T0384884

EMDR *and* PSYCHOTHERAPY INTEGRATION

Theoretical and Clinical Suggestions
with Focus on Traumatic Stress

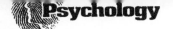

INNOVATIONS *in* PSYCHOLOGY

EMDR and
PSYCHOT
INTEGR

Theoretical and Clinic
with Focus on Trauma

How

C
Boca Raton   London

Library of Congress Cataloging-in-Publication Data

Lipke, Howard.
   EMDR and psychotherapy integration : theoretical and clinical suggestions with focus
on traumatic stress / Howard Lipke.
         p.   cm. — (Innovations in psychology)
   Includes bibliographical references and index.
   ISBN 0-8493-0630-2
   1. Eye movement desensitization and reprocessing. 2. Psychic trauma—Treatment.
I. Title. II. Series.
         [DNLM: 1. Desensitization, Psychologic—methods. 2. Combat Disorders—therapy.
   3. Eye Movements. 4. Psychological Theory. 5. Stress Disorders, Post-Traumatic—therapy.
   WM 425.5.D4 L764e   1999]
   RC489.E98L56   1999
   616.85'210651—dc21
   DNLM/DLC
   for Library of Congress   99-38186
                                                                              CIP

Series Preface

The first time I visited a Veterans Administration facility was after I had completed and published my first book *Stress Disorders among Vietnam Veterans: Theory, Research, and Treatment* (Figley 1978). The facility was a VA Medical Center in Indiana that specializes in mental health treatment. My guide at the facility explained that their role was more associated with "caring for the poor" than caring for those who "bore the battle."

Yet, I believed that it was the right thing to do, even though the nation was serving the health care needs of its poor under the guise of veterans services. I couldn't see why we were so confident that the care would be superior to the care of a neighborhood doctor. Back then, in the late 1970s, few therapists were familiar with combat-related PTSD. The diagnostic category was not invented until 1980, thanks to the American Psychiatric Association and its *Diagnostic and Statistical Manual of Stress Disorders* (1980). After publishing the findings of our interviews with Vietnam combat veterans, we produced *Strangers at Home: Vietnam Veterans since the War* (Figley and Leventman 1980). During that year, we helped establish the Readjustment Counseling Program within the VA; the Vet Center Program became a reality. It became one of the most successful programs in VA history because it was designed and applied for the exact purpose of doing something more than the neighborhood doctor could.

Even with the knowledge we gained in the 1970s and 1980s, a colleague of mine, who sees and treats war veterans all day long, looks back over his many years of experience and reports that his clients can be classified into three groups. He observes that about one third, Group A, gets better; another third, Group B, gets worse; and the final third, Group C, does not change. What must it be like to try, day in and day out, to help clients stay out of Group B or C and join those in Group A, who improve significantly? Those who do this often experience compassion fatigue, a form of burnout associated with resigning to the belief that clients will never get much better.

Eye Movement Desensitization and Reprocessing (EMDR) has given hope to good therapists who, like Dr. Howard Lipke, want to make a difference. They have found that EMDR is a category changer. EMDR has been studied more than any other treatment of the psychological effects of trauma, and the results show that EMDR treatment should be a priority.

Now comes this fine book by Dr. Lipke on the subject of EMDR and its role in psychotherapy in general and in trauma treatment in particular.

It has been 11 years since EMDR was introduced to the practice community. As editor of the *Journal of Traumatic Stress*, where Francine Shapiro published the first controlled research article on EMDR, I was struck by the enthusiasm, both negative and positive, of the reviewers. Two reviewers thought that a treatment approach that involved waving your hand in front of a client was sheer nonsense. Two other reviewers were quite excited and impressed with the results. Forty thousand trainees later, EMDR has been adopted more quickly by therapists than any other new psychotherapy approach. This was in large part due to Shapiro's ability to translate her clinical observations into an understandable approach that clarifies the life experiences the client wanted to review and clearly taps all of the aspects of the effects of the experience.

In his book, Dr. Lipke shares his considerable experience with the use of EMDR and helps readers translate and transcend their own paradigm to and from the EMDR approach. This book is about what he has learned about EMDR and its clinical use, particularly with combat veterans.

The heart of this important book is Lipke's Four-Activity Model, an extension of Shapiro's (1995) Accelerated Information Processing (AIP). Lipke offers a conceptual framework on psychotherapy in general by which to integrate Shapiro's theory on how dysfunctional memory can be reprocessed, provides the clinical findings on EMDR, and discusses the theory and findings of the broad range of other approaches to psychotherapy. This model also provides guidelines for practitioners in the use of EMDR. In providing these guidelines, Lipke applies his nearly 30 years of clinical experience using more traditional treatment approaches, along with his 10 years of using and teaching EMDR. It is an extension of, rather than an introduction to, EMDR.

The benefits of this book to practitioners working with distressed clients will quickly become obvious. Read it, and see what can now be done for our clients, veterans, and non-veterans suffering the effects of trauma.

Charles R. Figley, Ph.D.
Series Editor

Contents

Acknowledgments

First and most important, I want to thank my clients who are veterans. I remain grateful for their service to, and sacrifice for, our country. I have been honored and educated by their willingness to share their thoughts and feelings. I hope they can take some satisfaction in knowing that this book, which is the result of developments during our work together, may help others. I also wish to thank the many EMDR training participants I have worked with, and from whom I have learned much. Their willingness to share of themselves to learn for their clients reflects the highest standard of our profession.

My debt of gratitude to Francine Shapiro is immeasurable. I hope it is clear that this volume is essentially a commentary on her innovations, which have helped thousands of people. Special thanks also goes to Phil Casell, whose willingness to read an early version of the manuscript was most helpful in setting me on a more reasonable path. I have too much for which to thank William Zangwill. He suffered through many explanations of the ideas herein, as well as submitting to a reading of the manuscript and providing a thoughtful commentary on it. Thanks also to Steve Silver, who offered his considerable knowledge and wisdom in reviewing a later form of the manuscript, and in a very timely manner. I am grateful to Charles Figley for his encouragement to publish this book, and for his seminal contributions to almost every aspect of the current effort to provide professional psychological aid to trauma survivors. I am likewise thankful to Bob Tinker and Herb Fensterheim for their helpful comments on the sections I found most difficult to write.

Kathryn Conover did a sensitive and professional job of editing the manuscript; if any mistakes slip through, she cannot be held responsible. I would also like to thank Barbara Norwitz, Christine Andreasen, and the CRC staff, who have all been helpful to an often confused first-time author.

In addition to those mentioned above, all of whom worked directly on the manuscript, the work of many other contributors is recognized in the text. I would have liked to explicitly express my gratitude to all of my family, friends, and colleagues who contributed to this book in various other ways and who supported my position in writing it; unfortunately, according to my sister, the list would be both too long and not long enough. I think she is right. I can only hope that I will be forgiven by family, friends, and colleagues who are not mentioned by name. As my association with many of these people has been through organizational connections, I can at least include those: thank you to the staff of the Stress Disorder Treatment Unit and the psychology department of North Chicago DVA Medical Center; the faculty and students of the St. Louis University graduate school department of psychology, 1971–1976; and the EMDR Institute staff, facilitators, instructors, and participants in the Chicago EMDR study group.

Finally, thank you to my wife Lynn and our children, Nora and Aaron, who were still teenagers when I began to work on this book. They too often listened to me say, "I have to go work on the book," or watched me attend to some other project; then they lovingly welcomed me back.

*Dedicated
with love and gratitude
to my parents
Shainey and Leonard Lipke*

Introduction

In 1972 I was a second-year graduate student trainee in the psychiatric day hospital of the St. Louis Veterans Administration Hospital. During that year, I worked with only one client who identified himself as a Vietnam combat veteran. Later in my career I was informed by many Vietnam veterans, in less than polite terms, that so few came for help because they didn't want anything to do with government institutions after their experiences in Vietnam. Many who did come did not long pursue the services: they found them to be ineffective, frightening, or hostile. Some veterans were told to just forget about the war, others were treated as if they were schizophrenic or crazy (almost none who told me about this were schizophrenic, unless they had a type of schizophrenia that did not include thought disorder or blunted affect), or they were treated purely as drug addicts.

Partly because there were so few combat veterans seeking treatment where I worked, and partly for want of knowledge by the staff (not because of lack of compassion), there was no training specific to working with the problems of returning combatants. Therefore, I improvised with my first client. He was having nightmares over the death of a friend, killed by a Vietnamese "civilian." I asked my client to write a narrative of the event, and used a variation of systematic desensitization to try to help him live with the memory. I asked him to go through the script of the event using a relaxation exercise every time he felt his tension rising. As I recall, he dropped out of treatment after one or two sessions. He did not indicate that he felt any relief during the treatment. My first work with a combat veteran was a failure.

As my career evolved, I later met with combat veterans individually and in groups at an outpatient VA mental health clinic. Eventually, in 1987, I was appointed director of one of the few intensive inpatient programs for psychological work with combat veterans. I was appointed to the position because of experience, and acknowledgment that it was "my turn," not because of any marked improvement in my success rate at helping clients resolve combat-related psychological problems. I do not want to ignore or minimize the help my colleagues and I were able to offer. I believe our clients did find some comfort from attending the individual and group sessions, benefited from what they learned, and were aided by crisis intervention, but only a small minority found pervasive symptom relief.

My therapeutic orientation at that time could best be described as eclectic, with a cognitive behavioral emphasis. The inpatient program's approach was similar. The inpatient program had many elements of a therapeutic community. Treatment, individually and in groups, included Rational Emotive Therapy, assertiveness training, exposure, education about symptoms, and relaxation training. The interventions of therapists in daily unstructured groups and individual sessions included interpretations from the positions mentioned above, as well as from more dynamic positions. A variety of medications were prescribed; minor tranquilizers were excluded and major tranquilizers were rare.

Over the course of this work I came to believe that, while we could help stop deterioration of functioning, there was relatively little that psychotherapy could do to help combat veterans with long-standing PTSD to resolve symptoms. It seemed that the best we had to offer was the curative factor that appears on Irv Yalom's (1985) list as Universality — the knowledge that the veteran was not alone, that others also had similar painful experiences. I saw many clients come to our inpatient program thinking that they were alone in their pain. They judged themselves uniquely crazy, weak, and/or cowardly for having had problems, such as flashbacks, fearfulness, and rage, in civilian life after their military experience. There was some genuine relief that came from seeing that others had these problems, even if the problems continued. Because of our limited results, when I met with prospective clients to discuss possible admission, I told them that if they participated in the program they could expect to experience considerable psychological discomfort as they gained self-knowledge, but they could not expect their symptoms to change appreciably.[1]

It didn't take long to find this work — the exposure to the client's emotions of rage, guilt, and sadness, to the horrible events of war (even from this great distance), combined with my limited ability to help — destructively stressful. I began to have trouble sleeping several nights a week and I thought almost continually about the problems of the treatment program. I also, for a variety of reasons, believed I could not leave this assignment.

In 1990 I had been the director of the inpatient program for three years when I received a note from a friend and distinguished colleague who closely followed the scientific and professional literature. He sent me copies of articles by Francine Shapiro (1989a,b) about a new method of psychotherapy that reported one-session symptom relief for clients with PTSD. The method was then called EMD. His note read: "I thought you might find this article interesting. This has got to be one of the strangest methods ever devised for treating PTSD! That Wolpe finds it credible (see editor's note) [Wolpe's editorial note to the Shapiro article] is even more curious. Maybe it works!"(5/11/90)

---

1. It is now a generally accepted opinion that the inpatient PTSD programs, as originally constituted, were not clinically successful (Johnson 1997). At this writing, however, there is some data to suggest that even in programs where limited use of EMDR is made, clients do report some improvement (Silver, Brooks, and Obenchain 1995) and that where EMDR is provided intensively, results may be profound (Botkin et al. 1998).

I thought, in fact, that it might be more curious than effective. However, the reasons to take this method seriously outweighed its strange, inexplicable method of action and television-therapist type results.

The decision to further explore EMD was made for several reasons:

1. Our clinical results at the time: the program's clients were not realizing much improvement from the methods we had been trying. The one promising method we knew of highly structured, individually administered Direct Therapeutic Exposure. Despite reported statistically significant gains in some combat veterans (Keane et al. 1989), we did not use it regularly because it had not shown the kind of clinical significance in our efforts, or in research by others, that compensated for its aversiveness.

2. Published research: EMD was introduced with a flawed, but still a controlled study, in a reputable peer-reviewed journal (Shapiro, 1989a). In addition, a case study appeared in the *Journal of Behavior Therapy and Experimental Psychiatry* (Shapiro 1989b), with a footnote by the editor, the venerable Joseph Wolpe, testifying that he had used EMD to help a client progress who had reached the limit of effect with the well-established behavioral methods Wolpe had pioneered. Although this was only one case, it was an instance in which EMD had passed a most severe test, acknowledgment of its effectiveness by the originator of a competing, well-established method.

3. Verification of research results: because Shapiro had published the location of the agency where she did her work with combat veteran subjects, I was able to contact a staff member there. The staff member, who was a combat veteran, volunteered that he had been a subject, and that the method had helped him significantly with his combat-related problems. I also contacted a highly regarded professional colleague who worked in the San Francisco Bay area where Shapiro practiced. He reported that Shapiro's reputation there was acceptable.

4. Personal experience: a colleague, Dr. Al Botkin, volunteered to be a subject. We used the method to help him overcome the anxiety from a situation in which a family member had almost been injured. After one or two sets of eye movement, Al's anxiety, when he considered this event, disappeared.

5. The standards of the field: this factor almost demands its own volume; however, the next few paragraphs will have to do.

It is particularly interesting to examine the standards of the field of that ancient time, 1989, when Shapiro introduced EMDR, to the standards just a few years later where reviewers could question results that do not demonstrate psychophysiologic change in subjects (DeBell and Jones 1997). I began to offer EMD to clients based on knowledge gathered from two journal articles. At that time even academic critics of EMD acknowledged the appropriateness of the use of new methods in some clinical situations. Herbert and Mueser (1991), in criticizing the dissemination of EMD, wrote:

> The widespread dissemination of EMDR appears premature in view of the lack of scientifically adequate support for the technique. Historically behavior therapists have required such support as a condition for the adaptation of clinical strategies, while recognizing that the exigecies of clinical practice dictate that the competent clinician must sometimes use unproven methods, and that the clinical innovation is necessary for the field to progress. (p. 173)

While, in their subsequent praise of then-current methods, these authors did not seem to understand the PTSD treatment or EMD outcome literature very well, they did acknowledge the acceptance of the use of "unproven" methods, even by academic behavior therapists. The flexibility of the standards of even behavior therapy was demonstrated, as the Australian psychologist Gary Fulcher pointed out in a talk at the 1994 AABT Conference in Atlanta the observation that Systematic Desensitization was in use for 10 years based on case studies. Outside the realm of behavior therapy, psychoanalysis had been accepted as mainstream treatment without any controlled research.

Any of my supervisors have been pleased for me to use either behavioral or psychodynamic, or many other methods such as Gestalt therapy, hypnosis, etc., none of which had been tested with controlled studies with this population. The most frequently used modalities of treatment for combat-related PTSD were process and exposure-based group therapies. Interestingly, at the time I began using EMD, and still as far as I can tell, there is still not one controlled study isolating this type of group therapy and demonstrating its effectiveness in the treatment of combat-related PTSD. Critics of EMD(R) for several years after Shapiro began teaching it often decried her offering training in the method without first meeting their standards of demonstrated effectiveness (Herbert and Mueser 1995). However, at the time she began using and teaching EMD she, and EMD, were far ahead of the field's meager standards for clinical use and training in a method of psychotherapy.

To return to the circumstances of my initial use of EMDR: considering all the factors, it seemed more unethical to not try EMDR than to try it. So we did, offering it first to clients who were near the end of either a 60- or 90-day treatment program. If EMD did work as well as reported, then we wouldn't want to deprive these clients of the opportunity to benefit. The results of the session offered to the first five clients was published in the journal *Psychotherapy* (Lipke and Botkin 1993): our first client obtained almost immediate results, similar to those reported by Shapiro. This veteran, in the months he had been in the program, had participated actively, appeared well motivated to change, and had improved his general anger management, but overwhelming emotional arousal persisted when he contemplated major traumatic events: betrayal by an American officer and his own negative self-thoughts for perceived inadequacy in combat when he was slow to respond after being knocked down by an explosion. After 20 minutes of EMD this veteran could talk about the events calmly; he showed new insight into his own behavior, and he no longer was upset with himself. He still disliked the officer who betrayed him, but he was not overwhelmed with rage when talking about him.

This client had received 3 months of therapy without making a dent in his trauma response, yet after 20 minutes of brief conversation and a total of about 3 minutes of eye movement, his response to this trauma was, to all appearances, resolved. There was no conventional explanation for this result. If he were responding to demand characteristics, telling us that he was improved just because we wanted to hear it, then he was the first veteran in that program ever to do so. If the results were due to cognitive behavior therapy or hypnosis, or any other conventional method that EMDR "really" was, then I had, miraculously, become a great practitioner of whichever method accounted for the results. If the results were due to flooding, then I had been able to show excellent results in about seven and one half sessions less than usual without having to prompt the client, repeatedly reminding him of trauma-related stimuli, or help him achieve a relaxed state after the session. As wonderful as it was to help a client achieve this result, what happened with another client was more interesting.

Another of these five first veterans was a quiet man who did not speak much in individual or group therapy sessions. Unlike the first client, he had not been recently employed and his overall adjustment, in addition to problems directly attributable to combat trauma, were more profound. This client said that his worst traumatic experience had to do with the death of some civilians for which he believed he was responsible. As the EMD therapy session unfolded, this veteran first reported decreased anxiety, as had the first veteran. Suddenly, he became upset and asked that we stop treatment. He went out of the therapy room with another staff member to calm down. When he returned he said that, as he became more comfortable with the memory, he got scared. He believed that he had made a "spiritual deal" — that if he stopped suffering, retribution would be taken against his family for the wrong he believed he had done.

The notion that suffering can be an obligation, and that it sometimes had secondary gain qualities, is certainly not new, especially in work with combat trauma. However, I had never heard a combat veteran make the point so spontaneously, explicitly, and certainly, especially this client. This may have reflected my inexperience or a lack of clinical skill. Even if either of these deficiencies could explain the novelty of this experience for me, then at the very least it could be suggested that EMD was capable of educating backward clinicians.

That is the story of the beginning of my interest in EMDR. Like my clients who got the most out of our program when they discovered the universality of their problems early in their inpatient experience, I learned the most from

EMDR in the first week when I found out that the intrusive aspects of PTSD were potentially quickly and effectively resolvable, and that this method of resolution could also provide a deeper and more certain understanding of the elements contributing to the pain following trauma. Readers of this book who have used EMDR will likely find that, like me, the majority of what they will ever learn about the method is experiential and occurs quickly, but what there is to learn after that is still spectacularly interesting.

This book, then, is about what I have learned about EMDR and its clinical use, especially with combat veterans. It is also about what trying to understand how EMDR works has taught me about psychotherapy in general. That second lesson is what I call the Four-Activity Model (FAM) of Psychotherapy, which grows out of a concept Shapiro (1995) refers to as Accelerated Information Processing (AIP). Shapiro's AIP description gives name to the idea that learned psychopathology can be considered dysfunctional held information, including thoughts, emotions, sensations, and behavior, that can be modified more quickly than previously believed by most therapists. The Four-Activity Model is an attempt to conceptualize how psychotherapeutic activity can be used most efficiently to reprocess dysfunctional held material and thereby resolve psychological problems.

Finally, this book is about what psychotherapy in general has taught me about EMDR. Even in her early explanations of EMDR, Shapiro taught that it was an integrative method, that it relied on the lessons learned by years of clinical work using dynamic, behavioral, and humanistic methods. In this book I will attempt to elaborate on that relationship and offer specific therapeutic suggestions that will rely on the wisdom of previously established therapeutic methods, as well as the wisdom of past philosophical inquiry and religion. The book starts with EMDR, proceeds to try to describe how EMDR and other methods can be integrated into an overall model of psychotherapy, and then works its way back to the concrete practical integration of psychotherapy in general.

The second half of the book has a practical focus on examples that are created mostly from my experience working with combat trauma. I hope that readers will see how these examples of interventions are easily generalized to other learning-based problems.

This book is also specifically not something. It is not an introductory text to EMDR. Dr. Shapiro (1995) has written the definitive work. I hope there is enough basic information about EMDR so that the discussion of psychotherapy integration is clear; however, there is not enough information to learn to practice EMDR expertly. Therapists should expect that — just as with other methods — training with practicum supervision is necessary for competent practice. Experienced psychotherapists sometimes have a negative response to this strong recommendation because the standard of the field has for so long been to try out even complex new methods based on journal reports, or even word of mouth. This has generally been acceptable, but is no longer.

My experience in the training of hundreds of licensed practitioners has taught me that, even after several hours of instruction in the practicum, clinicians talk to clients when they should be asking them to move their eyes, and attempt to lead clients when they should be following them.

Shapiro has written the definitive manual on EMDR; however, in addition to attempting to add to Shapiro's work, I will occasionally make suggestions for minor changes in her protocols. These do not repudiate Shapiro's work but rather, I think, reflect the growth that comes with continued observation, by more clinicians working with different populations.

Much of this book is written in the first person. I often say, "I think this or that...." I hope this does not give the impression that I think I am the only person who ever had these thoughts, because I do fully and respectfully realize how much what I am writing has been thoroughly influenced by my predecessors and peers. I persist in the first person, not because I think I deserve credit, but because I do not want to claim false authority. I know that what I write are my thoughts based on the influences that have affected me, and may not be the revealed truth.

Having addressed all the other themes in the title of this book, and other matters that I believe needed to be clarified, I come to the last word in the title, the seemingly innocuous word *psychotherapy*. I am not comfortable with *psychotherapy* as a label to describe my professional activity of meeting with people to provide them with professional services. I dislike it so that I have toyed with the idea of borrowing from a popular musician, referring to it by symbol, and verbally calling it "the activity formerly known as psychotherapy." Granted that what I do has an effect on my clients' health, and that many of them have illnesses that include impaired brain or metabolic functioning. Yet I do not consider the medical model, illness cured by therapy, to be the best description of what I do any more than I would consider a hydraulic sanitation model used by industrial engineers and plumbers to be best described through the concepts of illness/diagnosis/therapy/cure, even though modern plumbing probably has more to do with health than all of our hospitals.

I agree with my colleagues who believe that "psychotherapy" is chiefly an educational/consultative activity. I prefer to consider myself, and ask my clients to consider me, a consultant who is trained to offer opinions and provide services concerning philosophical, emotional, behavioral, and interpersonal matters, similar to consulting a lawyer on legal matters. Unfortunately, some of my clients do not accept this type of relationship; they either prefer or are perhaps impelled to see me as having authority over them rather than as their employee. This is, of course, part of their problem and, again, not a part that would reasonably be considered medical.

Despite misgivings, I do use the words *psychotherapy* and *psychotherapist*, but I hope that in the near future another word that does not carry the same connotations can be found and widely accepted. I think the terms *counseling* and *counselor* had the potential to convey the concept, and I sometimes use them interchangeably with *psychotherapy* and *psychotherapist*. However, *counseling* is in common use with the restricted domain of marriage and career work. The best alternative I have been able to come up with is *emotional/philosophical consultant*. Obviously not catchy.

The reader may note that this is quite a thin volume, especially given the broad nature of the subject — the integration of all psychotherapy. My purpose here is to offer a framework and some clinical suggestions; I do not have the talent or time to fully elaborate on all the areas touched upon, only enough of each to establish credibility of direction. It is also my hope that readers who believe I have noticed something of worth here or there will pursue these matters more thoroughly.

In addition to the work involved in completing even a small volume, the major mental impediment in writing this book was the issue of privacy. I think of counseling as a restricted yet intimate relationship: restricted *because* it is so intimate. In therapy normal boundaries of disclosure are expanded, so unusual borders of time and place contact must be erected to protect the therapist and client from being totally enveloped by the relationship. Sharing what I have learned in such intimate relationships, although it does not violate confidentiality, brings uncomfortable feelings because a border of confidentiality is approached. I hope that my clients, though they are not identifiable from the vague and masked examples herein, will be pleased that some of what we have learned together is available to help others.

chapter 1

The Scientific Evidence and EMDR

A brief description of Eye Movement Desensitization and Reprocessing (EMDR) includes the following:

1. EMDR is a method of psychotherapy that engages clients in many traditional elements of other therapeutic methods, organized in a unique way.
2. As originally developed and most often practiced, the therapist has the client engage in episodes of moving his or her eyes back and forth, following the therapist's fingers.
3. Shapiro's initial research reported single-session resolution of long-standing, treatment-resistant psychological problems; subsequent research supports rapid treatment results.

I have learned from speaking publicly about EMDR that these three sentences introduce information that makes it almost impossible for me to proceed further, in an orderly way, to satisfy all of my audience. Some professionals, when informed that a method of psychotherapy involves therapist-directed eye movement, have a strong need to concretely understand the exact form this method takes before accepting any other information on the subject. Others will just as strongly, and justifiably, need to know that there is an empirical reason to take this claim seriously before they can make the effort to understand it further. A third group will insist on knowing that these claims are theoretically possible before further consideration. It is far easier to integrate the three kinds of information in verbal conversation than it is when writing. When speaking to an audience in person, one may use asides, tone of voice, and gestures to convey information on several channels at once. The immediate feedback enables one to tell which part of the message needs to be elaborated quickly; further, one can estimate the audience well enough to immediately respond to the most hostile group (challenging entrenched assumptions always has the potential to precipitate strong reactions).

When writing, a choice must be made and that is to bow to the empiricists and first demonstrate that EMDR is worth discussing. These skeptics have earned this bow, as it seems that the part of our nature that claims much and proves little has too often and too easily won out. In Chapter 2, I will address the theoretical underpinnings of the method, then get into the specifics: the jumping-off point to present my integrative model of psychotherapy.

EMDR Research Studies

The largest body of research on EMDR is in the treatment of Post-Traumatic Stress Disorder (PTSD). I will focus my review on the psychotherapeutic research in this area, which I believe supports the assertion that EMDR is the most effective method of treatment for the psychological effects of trauma. I will not try to defend the proposition that EMDR usually does this in one or two sessions of treatment. I think the "one session" success that Shapiro reported in her initial controlled study has resulted in more misconceptions and distracting criticism than any other aspect of EMDR.

In Shapiro's initial controlled study of EMDR, she treated 22 subjects mostly referred to her by a variety of mental health professionals, but included a few self-referrals — counselors in the participating agencies who wanted to work on unresolved trauma. It is essential to note that Shapiro's initial report only claimed that the subjects she treated were able to resolve a *single episode of trauma* in one session. This design, and therefore these results, cannot and should not be replicated. When Shapiro first used her method, following the standards of the day, she did not do extensive evaluation and explanation of the method. She had no reason to be concerned that other problems would arise because, in her experience, this had not happened. In addition, Shapiro used EMDR with an outpatient population that therapists were confident could be exposed to a novel treatment and an unknown therapist.

When I first tried EMDR it was not because I expected to replicate Shapiro's level of success; I only hoped to see if her results were credible. My clients had multiple trauma; they were inpatients in a system they mistrusted; and a mistaken diagnosis of mental health by therapists could lead to a loss of disability payments, thereby threatening personal and family survival.

While I realized my clients were different from Shapiro's, unfortunately some inexperienced colleagues working with clients who have similarly complex problems, or who have limited skill using EMDR, sometimes demand the rapid results of Shapiro's initial study when evaluating the credibility of EMDR. One example is that of Jensen (1994), who perhaps believed he was being charitable when he used two sessions of EMDR to treat chronic combat-related PTSD. Jensen reported small but significant changes in subjective distress related to the targeted traumatic memory, but no changes on a more global measure of mental health. In addition, Jensen applied the method poorly. Nonetheless, he and the editors of the prestigious journal *Behavior Therapy* appeared comfortable with Jensen's assertion that his study had helped to demonstrate that EMDR was not an effective treatment for PTSD.

Similarly and more recently, as reported in *Behavior Therapy,* Devilly, Spence, and Rapee (1998) found some positive results with EMDR in only two sessions, even on some global measures of PTSD, with combat veteran clients who had already received considerable treatment over many years. After finding this result in a difficult-to-treat, chronically symptomatic, multiply traumatized population, the authors nonetheless conclude that EMDR's efficacy is not supported. Multiply traumatized combat veterans with chronic severe symptoms of PTSD cannot be expected to make global mental health gains with one or two sessions, even if the sessions are successful.

With that said, I would like to leave the subject of holding EMDR to inappropriate tests of its effectiveness, and explore what I consider to be more relevant ways of evaluating EMDR's value.

The ideal strategy for judging the relative effectiveness of psychotherapy methods is head-to-head comparisons: subjects are randomly distributed to treatment and other controls are in place, such as blind and standardized evaluation of results. There are several published comparative studies of EMDR at this writing that meet many of the criteria of good research. Vaughn and associates (Vaughn et al. 1994) found positive results for all treatments when they compared EMDR to an exposure procedure and a relaxation procedure. However, EMDR showed a significant advantage because far less treatment time was used (the other treatment required daily homework) and EMDR better ameliorated intrusive symptoms.

In a study by Carlson and associates (Carlson et al. 1998) veterans with chronic combat-related PTSD were treated with EMDR or biofeedback for 12 sessions. Subjects receiving EMDR reported significant clinical and statistical pretreatment, posttreatment and follow-up improvement, as well as significantly better results than the biofeedback subjects on almost all measures. These included mean Mississippi Scale for Combat-Related PTSD scores decreasing from approximately 118 to posttest and follow-up results both below 95. Biofeedback subject scores went from 120 to approximately 115 at posttest, then approximately 113 at follow-up. The accepted cutoff for PTSD diagnosis with this test, which is not sensitive to change in subject condition, is 107 (Keane, Caddell, and Taylor 1988). Beck depression score results for the EMDR group began at approximately 20, decreased to below 10, and stayed there at follow-up; results for the biofeedback group went from about 23 to 16 at posttest, then up to about 18 on follow-up. Significant improvement was found on psychophysiologic measures for both treatment groups. Carlson concluded:

> Compared with other conditions, significant treatment effects in the EMDR condition were obtained at post-treatment on a number of self-report, psychometric, and standardized interview measures. Relative to the other treatment group these effects were generally maintained at 3-month follow-up. (p. 3)

Standardized instruments that yielded positive results favoring EMDR treatment included the Mississippi Scale for Combat-Related PTSD; the CAPS interview, including measures of reexperiencing combat trauma, avoidance, and arousal; and measures of anxiety and depression. On the other hand, one measurement of avoidance symptoms (a section of the IES scale) and the physiological indices of arousal did not yield effects differentiated by treatment.

Marcus, Marquis, and Sakai (1997) compared EMDR to standard care as the individual psychotherapy component of treatment provided to PTSD clients by an HMO psychiatric clinic. Subjects, randomly divided into treatment groups, were evaluated pretreatment, after three sessions, and on the completion of treatment (or at the end of the study; that is, 0.5 to 1 year, if treatment was not completed) by an independent evaluator. A variety of standardized measures were employed and demonstrated the EMDR subjects to improve significantly from baseline, and significantly more and more rapidly than the standard care group. Impact of Events scores for the EMDR group were 46, 25, and 18 at pretest, three sessions, and completion, respectively; standard care scores were 49, 47, and 35. Beck Depression Inventory scores for the EMDR group averaged 19, 13, and 8 at those time periods, while standard care scores were 22, 20, and 15. After three sessions, 16 EMDR subjects still met DSM-IIIR criteria for PTSD; 16 did not. After three sessions, 23 standard care subjects did and 6 did not. At completion, 7 EMDR subjects met PTSD criteria and 24 did not, while the standard care group split evenly on this measure, 16 and 16. While this study had the disadvantage of the control treatments was being standardized, it had the rare and valuable feature that therapist allegiance efforts, now being considered an important outcome study variable, were limited (Lubarsky et al. 1997).

Scheck, Schaeffer, and Gillette (1998) worked with female clients, 16 to 25 years old, recruited from local community service agencies. Inclusion criteria were dysfunctional behaviors such as sexual promiscuity, runaway behavior, substance abuse, and a self-reported traumatic memory. Ninety percent reported being victims of physical or emotional abuse as a child. Seventy-seven percent met criteria for diagnosis of PTSD. The 60 subjects were randomly assigned to two sessions of either EMDR or Rogerian supportive therapy, referred to as active listening (AL) to work on their most troubling memory. A variety of standardized measures were used to compare subjects; on all of these, EMDR demonstrated significant pre- and posttreatment differences, and outperformed the supportive counseling. Two measures included 90-day follow-up. On the Beck Depression Inventory, EMDR subjects' pre- and posttreatment and follow-up mean scores were 21/6/5; AL group scores were 26/16/14. On the Impact of Events scale, EMDR scores were 48/24/16; AL scores were 49/35/26. Results for subjects meeting full criteria for PTSD were not significantly different from scores for subjects not meeting full criteria.

Using a different design, Silver, Brooks, and Oberschein (1995) showed a statistically significant advantage for EMDR compared to relaxation biofeedback with difficult-to-treat patients — veterans with chronic combat-related

PTSD. The Silver study also showed EMDR to be more effective than relaxation training on several measures. A strength of the study was that the comparisons were made retrospectively, so that the type of expectancy effects naturally generated in prospective studies were not operative. (Of course, this meant that subjects could not be assigned randomly, a weakness of the study.)

Another source of comparison of EMDR with other methods is the judgment of therapists who have used EMDR, as well as other methods. This valuable resource has acknowledged weaknesses, but also strengths not easily found in any but the most expensive and time-consuming designs. One justification for examining the judgment of therapists is suggested by the work of Strupp and Hadley (1977; Strupp 1996), who offered three meaningful perspectives from which to evaluate psychotherapeutic effectiveness: the judgment of the client, of the society, and of the therapist. Another value, similar to that ascribed to the 1995 Silver study, is that the comparison is made based on work in the clinical setting, and is therefore highly generalizable. Obvious weaknesses, especially concerning control for expectancy effects, require that laboratory studies be done; however, once such studies are done and establish the basic effectiveness of a treatment extensive surveys can provide a wealth of information.[1]

In the survey of therapists relevant here, the first 1,295 clinicians trained by Shapiro in EMDR were questioned at least 7 months after their training. This extensive survey, looking for both positive and negative effects in a variety of areas, was returned by 407 subjects, or 31%. A follow-up mailing and a phone call were made to encourage participation of a randomly selected 10% of nonresponders; 35 therapists, 39% of that sample, returned surveys in response to those efforts. Thus, through direct and random sampling, 58% of the population have their opinions represented. The largest percentage of respondents, 49% to the first mailing, were licensed clinical psychologists. Of the second mailing, 29% fell in that category and 29% were licensed marriage and family counselors.

A series of questions were asked in the same format, with subjects given the choice of three answers: "More often," "As often," or "Less often." To the question, "Compared to other treatment methods you have used, how often have EMDR sessions led to general beneficial therapeutic effects?" 354 subjects in the first mailing responded; 76% found EMDR beneficial more often and 4% less often. In the second mailing, 70% found EMDR beneficial more often and 4% less often. To a similar question about "general negative side effects," of 326 first responders, 8% reported these "more often" with EMDR and 46% reported these "less often." Of the follow-up group, 4% reported these "more often" with EMDR and 30% "less often."

Because EMDR has so often been compared to flooding and implosion, even though the methods are very different (that is, EMDR instructions are

---

1. It also provides an empirically based clinical lore, in contrast to the traditional lore, which often consists of information as sound as urban myth.

to have the client just follow the content of consciousness after the target situation is introduced, while standard exposure continuously directs clients to target stimuli), the survey asked subjects who had "used imaginal [for example, flooding, implosion] exposure procedures" to compare EMDR and exposure on three dimensions: effectiveness, stressfulness to the client, and stressfulness to the therapist. There were four categories of answers: "EMDR more," "Equal effects," "EMDR less," and "Variable effects." On effectiveness, of 91 respondents, 57% reported "EMDR more" and 19% reported "EMDR less." On client stress, of 90 respondents, 11% reported "EMDR more" and 59% reported "EMDR less." On stress to the therapist, of 86 respondents, 21% reported "EMDR more" and 47% reported "EMDR less."

In summary, published studies comparing EMDR to other methods clearly favor EMDR for alleviation of the psychological effects of traumatic events.

Comparing Best Results with Best Results

Another way to use outcome data to examine the comparative effectiveness of EMDR is to compare the best results reported with EMDR to the best results reported with other methods of therapy. This approach takes into account the one usually unaddressed factor that pervades all evaluation of psychotherapy: *therapist competence* with the methods employed. As a field, we are more willing to address the question of training than the question of competence. There are many reasons for this, some related to the difficulty of doing science in this area, and some related to political or economic issues.

In comparing best results with best results, not every study on EMDR or other methods will be presented; I include only those that show the most positive outcome.

As a general framework for evaluating the best results of various treatments, we may consider Martin Seligman's (1993) authoritative (by way of his stature) popular press assessment of mental health treatments, in which he did not consider EMDR. He opens the chapter on PTSD by declaring "This is the saddest chapter of all." (p. 135) He concludes this chapter by stating, "Of all the disorders we have reviewed, PTSD is the least alleviated by therapy of any sort. I believe the development of new treatments to relieve PTSD is of the highest priority" (p. 144).

Combat-Related PTSD

It is possible to be more charitable to other treatments than Seligman suggests; Peniston and Kulkosky (1991) treated subjects with chronic combat-related PTSD with 38 half-hour sessions of Alpha/Theta Neurofeedback. They reported significant changes on the MMPI; had decreases in psychotropic medication use in 14 of the 15 subjects on medication. Without providing criteria, they indicated that at 30-month follow-up only 3 subjects relapsed.

In the realm of exposure procedures, Cooper and Clum (1989) used 6 to 14 sessions of flooding with 7 subjects with combat-related PTSD. They reported statistically and behaviorally significant changes on a number of variables. Beck Depression Inventory scores dropped from a pretest mean of 21 to a posttest mean of 12, and remained at 13 at 3-month follow-up. Nightmares declined from 3.1 per week to 0.1 at posttest and were at 1.2 on follow-up. However, average heart rate in response to a trauma provocative tape was essentially unchanged.

More recently, Frueh and associates (Frueh et al. 1996) treated 15 Vietnam veterans with chronic combat-related PTSD. They used a comprehensive treatment method that included 11 sessions of 90 minutes of exposure, plus a variety of other behavioral techniques to help with social relations and anger management. Treatment consisted of 29 individual and 90-minute group sessions. Results indicated significant improvement on a number of measures including Clinician Administered PTSD Scale scores (CAPS, pre x = 82.46, post = 65.55); heart rate when exposed to a script of a target trauma scene (pre x = 89.73, post = 77.00); and a number of other measures, including behavioral measures of nightmares (pre = 9.73/week, post = 5.55/week) and flashbacks (pre = 9.00/week, post = 6.27/week). Data on the Beck Depression Inventory and self-report anxiety and anger scales were simply reported as not significantly changed.

The most relevant EMDR study in this category is the 1998 Carlson study reported previously; ten veterans with chronic combat-related PTSD, treated with EMDR for 12 sessions, reported significant clinical and statistical improvement at least comparable to the above studies. Positive EMDR results have also been reported with this difficult-to-treat group by Boudewyns and Hyer (1996), who found significant changes in heart rate and the CAPS with five to seven sessions of EMDR, compared to "standard care" subjects who demonstrated no such change. Because this study is relevant to the role of eye movement in EMDR, it is considered more fully later, and only mentioned here to demonstrate that the Carlson et al. strong positive treatment results with combat veterans have been replicated.

Noncombat-Related PTSD

In a study of treatments of rape-related trauma, Foa and associates (Foa et al. 1990) compared three treatments and a no-treatment condition. Prolonged exposure (which included seven therapy sessions of listening to a narrative of the trauma for an hour, plus one listening per day as homework), was compared to Stress Inoculation Training (SIT, a variety of relaxation and cognitive behavioral procedures), and supportive counseling. Significant improvement was reported on several measures of symptomatology. In the exposure treatment condition, 9 subjects of the 14 who began treatment completed the study through the 3-month follow-up. Beck Depression Inventory scores for these subjects averaged 15.1 pretreatment, dropped to 12.7 posttreatment, then dropped to 6.4 on follow-up. In the SIT group, 9 of

14 subjects who completed through follow-up scored 21.4 at pretest, 6.8 at posttest, and 10.3 on follow-up. The pre, post, and follow-up scores for the supportive counseling group were 21.4, 19.0, and 15.9, respectively. Less impressively for the exposure and SIT method, Foa and associates reported that at follow-up 45% of the exposure and Stress Inoculation Training subjects still met criteria for PTSD, while not many more, 55%, of the supportive control subjects met criteria for PTSD. (The difference was one subject per group.)

Resick and Schnicke (1992) studied Cognitive Processing Therapy (CPT), described as a combination of education, exposure, and cognitive therapy, in the treatment of rape-related PTSD symptoms in subjects without "severe competing pathology." Treatment consisted of 12 1.5-hour sessions (including two exposure sessions) with homework added. Of the 19 subjects, 17 met full DSM-IIIR criteria for PTSD. At the 6-month follow-up, only 2 of the 16 available subjects met criteria. Impact of Event Scale scores dropped from 42 to 18 from pretest to follow-up. Beck Depression Inventory scores declined from 21 to 10 over this time period.

Echeburua and colleagues (1996) treated 20 victims of sexual assault who met DSM IIIR criteria for PTSD. The study compared the effectiveness of "cognitive restructuring and specific coping skills training" with progressive relaxation training for treatment-seeking subjects. Each group received five 1-hour sessions. Pre, post, and follow-up results were impressive. Most gains for both groups, on a structured PTSD interview and several standard measures, took place by the end of treatment with improvement continuing for both groups through the follow-up. The cognitive intervention group did significantly better and showed substantially more follow-up improvement. By 1-month posttreatment, none of the cognitive treatment group was diagnosed with PTSD, while at 1 month five relaxation subjects were not diagnosable and only eight met this criteria at one year. An example of change magnitude is exemplified by the Beck Depression Inventory mean scores, which were 20/9/4 at pre/post/1 year for the cognitive group and 18/8/4 for the relaxation subjects. While the level of success for these treatments is very high, the role of the treatments in contributing to it is tempered by three facts: subjects were treated, on average, 5 weeks posttrauma; subject selection criteria excluded those "affected by other syndromes" (other than acute PTSD); and the therapist administered the measures of treatment effects. The length of time between trauma and treatment is relevant because it has been noted that there is considerable symptom relief for a substantial proportion of sexual trauma victims during the 4 months following the assault (Rothbaum et al. 1992).

Figley and Carbonell (1995) have reported preliminary results in a study of a variety of PTSD treatments. One notable finding was significant improvement in Subjective Units of Disturbance scores (SUDs) following extremely brief treatment with Thought Field Therapy (TFT), a procedure introduced by Roger Callahan. Although the report of study results was limited, and subject inclusion criteria were not well specified, positive findings and brevity of treatment suggests TFT may be a promising method.

In the only quantitatively measured study I could find on the methods in the treatment of PTSD, Brom, Kieber, and Defares (1989) reported statistically significant improvement for subjects treated with hypnotherapy, trauma desensitization (a variation of systematic desensitization), and brief dynamic psychotherapy. While reports were positive, posttest Impact of Events Scale results indicated marked continuing symptom presence.

The non-EMDR "best" results discussed above may be compared to EMDR "best results." Renfrey and Spates (1994), in studying the role of eye movement in EMDR treatment of PTSD symptoms, treated 16 of their subjects with standard EMDR techniques. (A comparison with the nonstandard technique will be addressed later, in the discussion of the role of eye movement.) Subjects showed heart rate reactivity to trauma stimuli declines of 8 beats per minute. Of 15 subjects who met criteria for PTSD before treatment in the standard eye movement conditions, only 2 met criteria after two to six sessions. These subjects' mean Impact of Events scores declined from approximately 30 to approximately 11 at follow-up. In addition to changes in measures of psychopathology, Renfry and Spates' subjects also, on a modified validity of positive cognition scale, improved their validity rating of positive self-statements from approximately 2/10 to above 8/10. This measure, suggesting positive information processing, is impossible to compare to results from other studies because other research has not examined measures of positive functioning.

In a study of 80 subjects, 3 months to 54 years posttrauma (half in a delayed treatment control), who received up to three 90-minute EMDR sessions, Wilson, Becker, and Tinker (1995) also found statistically and clinically significant results treating traumatic memories and PTSD. Impact of Event score means decreased from above 30 at pretest to below 10 at posttest and remained at that level at 3-month follow-up. The delayed treatment group was essentially unchanged on the IES. State-trait Anxiety Index and Symptom Checklist-90-R subtest scores dropped in a similar manner. These improvements were maintained for the 61 subjects who were available at 15-month follow-up (Wilson, Becker, and Tinker 1997). At the beginning of the study, 37 Wilson subjects met all five DSM-IV criteria for PTSD and 17 were sexual molestation or rape victims. Statistical analysis was reported to indicate that improvement was not related to whether or not criteria for PTSD were met, type of trauma, or any other easily identifiable variable, other than the presence of EMDR treatment. At the 15-month follow-up only 4 of the 29 responders who initially met all criteria for PTSD still met diagnostic criteria.

Finally, Rothbaum (1997), a coauthor of the Foa et al. (1991) study, compared EMDR to waitlist control for 21 rape victims who met DSM-IIIR criteria for PTSD, and were treated at least 3 months posttrauma. Three dropped out during assessment; thus, ten subjects were treated and eight were in waitlist group. Treatment consisted of three therapy sessions. Rothbaum reported that "only one EMDR subject (10%) met full criteria for PTSD at posttreatment, compared to 88% of control subjects." On the Impact of

Events Scale, EMDR subjects scored 47/12/6 at pretest/posttest/follow-up, while control subjects scored 49/45 at pretest/posttest. On the Beck Depression Inventory, EMDR subject scores were 21/7/8 at pretest/posttest/follow-up, while waitlist subjects were 35/30 at pretest/posttest.[2] EMDR subjects performed better on a wide variety of measures, achieving statistically significant differences on most — but differences that were not significant on some, such as the Dissociative Experiences Scale; on the latter, EMDR subjects scored 25/12/8 at pretest/posttest/follow-up and waitlist subjects scored 30/23 on pretest/posttest. Rothbaum reported that waitlist subjects, when later offered EMDR, performed comparably to the initial EMDR subjects.

Does the comparison of "best results" of EMDR treatment with "best results" of other treatments demonstrate that EMDR is a distinct and efficacious form of therapy? I believe the evidence is reasonably convincing that it does. While some non-EMDR methods report substantial therapeutic gains, the best EMDR results appear to surpass the best of each of the other treatments on at least one of the following dimensions: power of therapeutic effect, brevity of treatment, difficulty of problem or population treated, and/or replication of results, while at least equaling the others on the other dimensions. Reviews of the literature on EMDR have sometimes faulted EMDR for not having treatment results that are demonstrable by objective measures (Lohr et al. 1995). This objection appears to have been met. In addition, the number of subjects treated with EMDR for PTSD symptoms far surpasses the number of subjects treated by exposure and other long-established treatments.

The results reviewed here strongly indicate that further consideration of EMDR as a method of therapy and its relationship to other methods are worth pursuing. The analysis is also consistent with a metaanalysis conducted by Van Etten and Taylor (1997, 1998), who summarize their results:

> As noted, EMDR and behavior therapy were the most effective psychotherapies, and both were generally more effective than SSRI treatments. Effect sizes were large across all PTSD symptom domains for both treatments, and treatments were statistically comparable in efficacy. Minimal differences in treatment efficacy between these treatments were noted across the various PTSD symptom domains. EMDR tended to be more effective than behavior therapy in treating depression and anxiety, and produced large effect sizes for these measures where behavior therapy produced only

2. The large difference between the pretest Beck Depression Inventory scores of the EMDR and waitlist groups suggest that these subjects may have been fundamentally different, which could modify the interpretation of the effect of treatment. However, when the waitlist group was finally given EMDR, BDI scores were also reduced, suggesting that EMDR is not limited in effectiveness when subjects have high initial BDI scores.

moderate effect sizes. Although both treatments maintained effects at follow-up, EMDR tended to increase
at follow-up, whereas behavior therapy effects remained stable, but did not increase notably. Moreover,
EMDR treatments entailed less therapy (5 vs. 15 hours)
over a shorter time period (4 vs. 10 weeks) in comparisons to behavior therapy. (1997: p. 17)

On to some theoretical discussion.

chapter 2

Accelerated Information Processing

EMDR was developed as a clinically integrative method of therapy, rather than as a theoretically integrated method. I will elaborate later, but one may easily see key features of Rational Emotive Behavior Therapy, experiential therapies, client-centered, dynamic, and other approaches. Shapiro has noted, even emphasized, that the development of EMDR was not theoretically based. She discovered that rapid, repetitive eye movement had a powerful anxiety reduction effect (initially attributed to desensitization); then, based on experience, she developed a therapeutic approach to accompany this discovery.

Developing a Theoretical Construct

Only after Shapiro developed EMDR and noted its effects in her work and the work of others did she put forward a theoretical construct, accelerated information processing (AIP), to provide a framework for the consideration of EMDR, as well as other methods of treatment which might share some of EMDR's properties.

There are many elaborate ways to discuss information processing as a theoretical position, and in a moment we will come to some of these. First, I would like to clarify what I mean by information processing. By *information processing psychology*, I mean that information, usually in the form of sensation or perception, is taken in by a person, it interacts with the person, change occurs, and usually at some point there is an output of activity, such as language or other behavior. At this stage of discussion there are no presuppositions about the nature of interaction between the person and the new information. (Although this is an obvious point I want to be explicit in taking information processing out of the realm of only verbal and visual psychology.)

Given acceptance of this broad input–throughput–output model, the next step is fraught with potential controversy. That is to specify the exact

nature of the elements and their interaction. There has been much sophisticated writing on this subject (for example, Barnard and Teasdale 1991;
Horowitz 1998; McClelland 1995). Much current information processing
thinking about psychopathology and psychotherapy in the behavior therapy
literature comes through Peter Lang's (1983) writing on fear-based psychological problems. Lang does not specifically consider PTSD, but Chemtob
et al. (1988) and Foa et al. (1989) do elaborate this line of thought.

According to information processing conceptualizations, we may look at
the experience-based part of psychopathology as coming from the thoughts,
feelings, visual images, behavior patterns — in short, the representation of
experience being stored in the brain — in a dysfunctionally, incompletely
processed manner. Lang refers to the components (thoughts, feelings, etc.) as
stimulus, response, and meaning propositions. It appears that he refers to the
information being held as propositions because it is held in parts and is
modifiable. These propositions are organized to form (in Lang's terms) *images*,
but will be referred to in most of this book as *networks*. The term *image* should
not be confused with mental pictures. The image, or network, of a death in
battle would contain many propositions. The stimulation of one aspect, or
proposition, in this network could activate the whole network and result in
a full reexperiencing of the event; alternatively, only part of the image, just
the fear, might be activated. Given this, "...the aim of therapy," Lang states,
"could be described as the reorganization of the image unit in a way that
modifies the affective character of its response elements." To this I would
add that the reorganization or reprocessing that occurs comes from a merging
of previously separated information networks, or the integration of the
"problem" network and newly introduced information.[1]

To this notion that networks consist of component parts, we also may
add the proposition, which Chemtob et al. (1988) summarize nicely, that the
components are arranged hierarchically and in subsystems. Thus, in a therapeutic context, if a client's PTSD network includes the belief that he is
cowardly, even if no running from danger was involved in his particular
trauma, a pathologically strong response may occur if he sees a film of people
running from danger, because running in fear is a behavior subsumed in the
hierarchy by the concept of cowardliness. After successful treatment that
allows the client to no longer define himself as a cowardly person, the same
film may not trigger a strong negative emotional response, even if the image
of people running from danger was never overtly addressed in therapy.

---

1. More recently Lang, Craske, and Bjork (1999) have summarized a position they report is
based on work by Bouton, and the theories of Bjork and Bjork, also written about by Foa and
McNally, that fear networks are not so much modified. Rather, in the extinction process, a new,
not-fear network supersedes an old fear one when it becomes more easily retrieved. By this
view, treatment is successful when the new associations are established and easily enough
retrieved to make the new response pervasive. This point of view explains why previously
extinguished responses may come back full force in some situations. Whether or not connections
within an "old" fear network are ever truly broken is an important point, not yet resolvable.
The standard practice of EMDR would not be changed by the implications of either model.

It should be noted here that, despite the hierarchical arrangement in which one might expect initiating change at the top would be the most efficient clinical work, the changing of the content of these networks begins at a concrete and specific level. For example, it does little good to work with self-esteem, an item at the top of the hierarchy, in the abstract. Clinical experience has taught me that it is ineffective to have an "expert" try to convince a person he should think better of himself. At least one specific event, and at least some of its concomitant specific thoughts, feelings, visual images, and self-statements, must be accessed first. As EMDR practice has shown change there can spread quickly to the highest levels of abstraction, but change begins at the lower level (see clinical examples in Chapter 3, the section on Category 3 activity). It seems there are internal laws of evidence that make clinical interventions at the level of the specific more compelling than expert testimony to a person's worth. The foundation of the general in the concrete, at even a semantic level, is interestingly demonstrated by Skinner (1989, 1990) in *American Psychologist* papers, where he traces the origin of words describing feelings, states of mind, and cognitive processes to the causes of the feeling; that is, to some aspect of behavior or to the setting in which the behavior occurred.

My invoking Skinner here does not mean that I endorse the notion that behavior is primary or the only aspect of experience that should be considered; rather, for experience-based (learned) psychological problems, the root is found in some aspect (thoughts and/or feelings, etc.) of specific events that may best be accessed through the concrete. Just as the word *agony* comes from a Greek word for a specific activity, "a struggle for victory in the games" (compact edition of the *Oxford English Dictionary* 1984), a client's pain may be most easily referenced or accessed through the concrete memory of a specific frustration, struggle, gunshot, or other event in the war or traumatic event.

It is important to make note that in information processing conceptualizations of psychopathology, it is experience-based problems that are being referred to. The distinction between experience and other psychological problems is made clear by Chemtob et al., who proffer a comprehensive explanation of the variety of PTSD problems. In their work, they allude to the idea that people who are highly susceptible to PTSD may be constitutionally prepared to develop conditional fear responses and resistance to extinction. If this is true, psychotherapies based on information processing might be expected to lead to decreased negative emotional response to given stimuli, but not to affect the underlying propensity to develop conditional fear responses.

In discussing therapeutic interventions to experience-based psychological problems, Lang includes exposure treatments, flooding, implosion, and systematic desensitization, but does not neglect the possible benefits of modeling or even components of "talk therapies." While he believes the ultimate goal of therapy may be to reduce the affective component, he seems to recognize that curative effects may come from changing other aspects of the network.

So what we have in the pre-accelerated information processing model is the recognition that experienced-based psychopathology is held hierarchically, in component parts, in networks that encompass many different aspects of experience, including "meaning." These networks, thus the experience, may be modified by a variety of therapeutic modalities; however, in order to be modified, the network — especially its affective components — must somehow be accessed.

Shapiro's AIP conceptualization starts with the premise common to other information processing models: learning-based psychopathology is the result of affectively painful emotion and other "negative" information held in the nervous system. She asserts that this is a dysfunctional state of affairs brought on by the blocking of normal information processing activity. She makes it clear that the goal of psychotherapy is not simply to decrease the negative emotion attached to events, but to thoroughly reprocess events so that the affect that accompanies memory of them may even be positive and the self-referent beliefs associated with the events are neutral at worst. Thus, AIP is distinguished by the beliefs that information is normally processed to an adaptive state unless it is blocked, and that removing the block(s) will result in positive adaptation.

A second distinguishing, and more revolutionary, feature derived from Shapiro's clinical work is that adaptive reprocessing can take place rapidly. Specifically, painful nonadaptive emotion, self-beliefs, and intrusive content, defined as part of psychopathology, can be resolved and traumatic events can often be positively integrated with the same speed that such maladaptive elements can be acquired.

The first notable quality of AIP — that adaptive functioning naturally follows the removal of a block — is not without precedent. In fact, it may be seen as an information processing interpretation of the Humanistic psychotherapeutic position asserted by Carl Rogers. The most striking assertion of the AIP model is that severely and chronically dysfunctional associative networks can be essentially, positively, and lastingly modified in minutes. The research cited demonstrates this fact empirically. This finding begs for a theoretical explanation, especially in light of recent persuasive research suggesting that associations formed based on extreme fear are permanent alterations in the nervous system (LeDoux 1992).

How EMDR Might Work

The first component of the explanation is the introduction of the idea that long-term memory can be divided into two types, declarative and nondeclarative, a distinction well summarized by Larry Squire and his associates (1987). *Declarative memory* contains facts, ideas, things that we know that we know. *Nondeclarative memory* refers to a variety of processes, including what we know as habituation, simple classical conditioning, and fixed behavior patterns (such as the coordinated movements of a refined golf swing).

Some information is retained in nondeclarative memory systems and some in declarative systems, and much is held in both.

Consider learning to play a tune on a piano as a way to integrate these concepts. When a novice player is first learning the tune, the notes are thought of consciously, narratively, one by one by their names: declarative memory is being used. With repetitive practice the tune comes out rapidly, the notes are no longer considered one at a time, but in bunches: at this point, nondeclarative processes dominate while the tune is being played. After playing "automatically," using nondeclarative processes, if the pianist wants to teach someone else, he may have to observe himself playing the tune to access the narrative instructions and convey them to another student.[2]

Information that contains strong negative emotional components may be initially taken into nondeclarative memory and not be well integrated into declarative systems. A frequent observation in traumatized individuals is the inability to recall much or any detail of traumatic events, while reacting emotionally to reminders of these events. Many clinicians have then noted that, as the client goes through successful treatment (that is, emotional upset is reduced), details of the traumatic event are consciously recalled. We may view this as the shift of trauma-related information from nondeclarative to declarative memory.

That the voluntary rapid bilateral eye movement found in the beginning incarnation of EMDR might have a role in this shift is suggested by research on spontaneous eye movement in information processing in general. Amadeo and Shagass (1963) presented results that suggested EM was significantly more frequent when subjects performed arithmetic than when they rested, and that the limiting of EM appeared to interfere with arithmetic ability. Studies performed by Antrobus et al. (1964) suggested EM is associated with the change of material in consciousness and problem solving. Ehrlichman and Barrett (1983), in reviewing this, other, and their own experimental data, propose that eye movement rate is reflective of cognitive change, especially in "…'sampling' many different contents, operations, or memory locations." This view of the role of eye movement suggests that the therapeutic benefit may be in directly activating the search for new ways of understanding the events under consideration.

A related hypothesis that could be supported by the cited work, as well as a line of research studied and discussed by Irwin and Carlson-Radvansky (1996), is that while the eyes are engaged in saccatic movement, thoughts — especially mental imagery — are suppressed. In this hypothesis, the brief suppression of aspects of the accessed associative network containing the target material allows previously unconnected material to come to the fore

---

2. Because psychotherapy for trauma primarily involves, according to this conceptualization, moving material from nondeclarative to declarative systems, one may get the impression that nondeclarative memory is maladaptive or that movement from nondeclarative to declarative is the norm. As may be gathered from the piano example, the adaptiveness of movement of memory depends on the task and the situation.

and become integrated with the associative network containing the target material. (See also Andrade et al. 1997, reviewed in Chapter 3.)

To go a speculative step further, it may be that this process takes place normally during sleep, especially during REM-stage sleep. Several researchers consider this stage of sleep to be the time in which the brain integrates information, especially emotionally powerful information (Cartwright 1991; Winget and Kapp 1972).

So if, as my clients have uniformly reported, they wake up in the dreams recounting trauma in the middle of events, not when they have reached safety, it may be speculated that the natural curative process has not been allowed to complete. Thus, traumatic material would remain stored primarily in nondeclarative memory, and retain the strong negative conditional components in the associative network.

One aspect of this explanation can easily lead to one being sidetracked: the fact that both EMDR and REM sleep contain rapid eye movements. This may be just a coincidence, since a variety of physical activities can be substituted for EM in EMDR. I think the most promising explanation for the role of EM (as discussed earlier) or other physical activity in the EMDR process is that the activity produces what is called an "orienting response" that precipitates psychophysiological activity which either promotes or allows the completion of information processing. (The orienting response will be discussed in slightly more detail in the next chapter.)

The role of EM has been controversial for several reasons, but the most disappointing one is the concrete interpretation by some researchers (Pitman et al., 1996): since EMDR is named after eye movement, it must stand or fail as a treatment only if the eye movements are the critical feature. These researchers somehow fail to note that Shapiro reported early in her work that other activities could substitute for eye movement.

To return to the question of rapidity of response, if one uses a traditional learning theory model with exposure-based treatments, it is difficult to fathom how therapeutic change can take place so quickly. However, when one switches to an information processing model herein, through which the therapeutic process facilitates use of natural integrative functioning rather than simple extinction processes, then rapid change is more readily comprehensible.

Lang et al. (1983) have pointed out that the first step in changing a network is to access it. It is difficult to define exactly what is meant by accessing. It is tempting to define it as "bringing to consciousness"; however, most networks contain too much information to be brought to consciousness at once. Perhaps accessing might better be seen as having the network partially in consciousness, with no aspect of it so strongly inhibited from consciousness that it leads to an attempt to block further awareness. According to conventional learning theory and years of clinical research, repetitive accessing of the negative conditional stimuli without presentation of the aversive event will lead to a decrease of the negative conditional response; likewise, the repeated pairing of the negative conditional stimulus with a positive unconditional response will also diminish the negative conditional response. What we may have found with EMDR is that conditional responses can change without repetitive trials more easily than previously thought.

It is recognized that complex and specific information processing models have been delineated to describe the paths through which the various types of information are processed or fail to process. It has not been my intention to describe these or to offer my own, beyond the observations described above. Those models, by theoreticians such as Lang, Chemtob, or Barnard and Teasdale, among others, describe the processes in detail unnecessary here. What is important, I think, is to recognize which phenomena must be accounted for. For our purposes, we don't need to know how exactly a scent may lead to partially reexperiencing a past event — only that there must be a connection that sometimes leads to this result. Likewise, we don't have to hypothesize the details of an exact system that explains how lasting desensitization to traumatic stimuli could follow either a set of eye movements or 12 sessions of exposure; we only have to acknowledge that both phenomena coexist. The simplified version of an information processing model and accelerated information processing offered here is designed to allow for what has been observed or appears to be logical necessity. To give another specific example, I don't try to account for how cognition and affect are connected, or whether or not connections can be completely erased; I only recognize that they may elicit each other at times and that, just as the connection can be formed, it *appears* as though it can be broken — not simply suppressed.

Whether this appearance of a broken connection is a rapid masking of an indelible classically conditioned emotional response, or partial (or full) severing of the connection, awaits further research.

Using the AIP theoretical position as a base, I will next describe EMDR in more detail and then offer an overall conceptualization of psychotherapy that allows for the integration of various methods, including EMDR.

chapter 3

EMDR and the Four-Activity Model of Psychotherapy

The Basics of EMDR

As promised, I will now describe the practice of EMDR as Shapiro introduces it in her text and workshops. Then, I will attempt to more fully integrate EMDR, the principles of AIP, and psychotherapy in general, into another theoretical framework, which I call the four-activity model of psychotherapy.

As Shapiro introduces EMDR, it is sometimes a freestanding method of psychotherapy and sometimes a portion of an overall psychotherapeutic strategy. In an established therapy relationship, some of the activities described will already have been accomplished and the reprocessing stage can begin more quickly. As a freestanding method to address the effects of a traumatic event, it contains eight phases.

History and Treatment Planning

Comprehensive evaluation and assessment are necessary to establish client goals and determine whether EMDR is an appropriate form of treatment. If it is, the client is educated about EMDR sufficiently to make an informed choice about accepting the treatment. Potential targets of reprocessing are selected, based on past and present experience and concerns about the future.

Preparation

This step further establishes the therapeutic alliance and gives more comprehensive information about EMDR and other treatment. Procedures are established to help the client manage possible increased distress. Obvious possible secondary gain issues are also explored in this stage.

Assessment

Not to be confused with general evaluation and history taking, at the assessment stage, the client identifies:

1. The target picture that represents the worst moment of the target event or some aspect of the event that symbolizes it
2. Present (negative) accompanying cognitions[1]
3. Desired (positive) alternative cognition that the client prefers to have accompany memory of the target event
4. Level of validity of the desired cognition (VoC)
5. Emotions present as the picture is accessed
6. Level of emotional distress (SUD rating) experienced as the image is reimagined and the emotions are attended to
7. Accompanying physical sensations

Desensitization

In this phase, the client focuses on the target picture and its attendant negative cognition, emotions, sensations, then begins a series of therapist-led lateral eye movements or substitute activities. This continues either until desensitization is achieved or the process is stopped for other reasons. During this stage, the therapist may also need to redirect client focus. The nature of this redirection is the content of the later clinical section.

Installation

When desensitization is achieved, the initially developed positive cognition or, if it has emerged, a better cognition, is paired with eye movement.

Body Scan

Following apparently complete processing, as indicated by no spontaneously noticeable discomfort, the client is asked to focus on the body, moving the length of the body, and notice any residual sensation.

Closure

Near the end of the time for the session, the therapist debriefs the client, especially discussing the possibility that new material may come to awareness. Keeping a journal of concerns and new material is encouraged.

Reevaluation

This phase involves the reassessment of the previous session's target material at the beginning of the next session.

1. In the broad sense, *cognition* includes the picture (visual image). Here, as in Shapiro's work and the traditions of cognitive therapies, the word *cognitive* is restricted to beliefs.

I believe that these eight phases of EMDR, as well as the activities of other methods of psychotherapy, can be conceptualized as containing up to four basic therapeutic activities. These activities may be seen as building blocks that may each take many forms, but do make up the universe of therapeutic activities. Before I get into the specifics of these activities, it may be important to address metatheories of psychotherapy in general.

The Integration of Psychotherapies: Metatheories

Since early in the history of psychotherapy, psychotherapists and personality theorists have interpreted the various schools and approaches of psychotherapy in their own terms. A classic example is Dollard and Miller's (1950) interpretation of psychoanalysis in learning theory terms. Similarly, psychoanalysts could view any positive therapeutic effects in psychotherapy in analytic terms — for example, referring to rapid gains as transference cures. In fact, any comprehensive theory of psychotherapy must be able to explain the findings of other psychotherapies in its own terms. Because these theories can, if they are going to remain viable, subsume other theories, they can also be considered metatheories. These theories (simultaneously, metatheories) of psychotherapy derived from the philosophical leanings, clinical findings, and experimental results of their respective founders.

There is another, more recently evolved, type of metatheory that derives from the study of methods of psychotherapy. This type of metatheory attempts to distill the findings of practitioners of the various methods into a set of active ingredients or key factors. Some of these metatheories are descriptive, such as Jerome Frank's (Frank and Frank 1991), aimed at describing similarities in previously established methods; others offer their own synthesized (integrationist) method, such as the Transtheoretical approach of Prochuska, Norcross, and DeClementi (1994), Arnold Lazarus' Multimodal Behavior Therapy (Lazarus 1989, 1992) and Psychosynthesis (Assagioli 1965).

The metatheory or, perhaps more accurately, *metamodel* that will be introduced here is descriptive. A new method of treatment is not introduced; rather, the insights obtained from the success of EMDR are used to reconceptualize the psychotherapeutic enterprise in general. I have found this reconceptualization useful in teaching and clinical work. It appears to reduce confusion when confronting the widely accepted view that psychotherapists of different theoretical schools have far more in common than they do that differentiates them in their actual practice.

Through this model, the seemingly disparate traditional methods of psychotherapy can be compared, contrasted, and integrated with accelerated information processing methods such as EMDR.

Introduction to the Four-Activity Model

We will return to EMDR or, more specifically, the parts of EMDR that are most unique and in which the bulk of therapeutic change takes place:

stages 3, 4, and 5: Assessment, Desensitization, and Installation. In the least complex cases, these phases can be seen as containing two therapeutic activities:

1. Accessing target associative networks
2. Processing the accessed material

We may simply call these activities *accessing* of material already stored in the mind and further *processing* (connection and transformation) of that material. Oftentimes, simply alternating between accessing and processing is all that is needed for successful resolution of a problem. The task is made even easier by the fact that processing often automatically leads to the accessing of the succeeding material to be processed.

Here is a simple general example, not uncommon, for a combat veteran. This client has a disturbing memory in which he believes he did not act courageously enough because he delayed the necessary moment before firing in a critical situation:

THERAPIST (*recapitulating the client's earlier responses*): Bring up a picture of the most disturbing moment of the battle, the thought, "I'm a coward," the anger and other emotions and feeling in your body, and follow my fingers. (*Therapist then leads client in set of EM.*) What comes to awareness now?

CLIENT: I did fire my rifle. I didn't run.

THERAPIST: Start with that. (*Therapist initiates another set of EM.*)

The client, in processing the initial image of perceived cowardice, accessed a new target for further processing: "I didn't run."

The two other categories of activity, as well as more sophisticated accessing, are used in EMDR in more complex situations. These two additional categories are the introduction of new information and the inhibition of accessing. In the example of the veteran who calls himself a coward, if he does not progress in processing the event to an adaptive conclusion just through accessing and processing, it may help him to learn that some delay in reaction is a biological limitation — he may not know this.[2] If the therapist introduces this information, during successive sets of EM the client may integrate the idea that his reaction was normal, not cowardly.

The final category of activity, the inhibition of accessing, is most often used when processing cannot be completed within a session. In this case the

2. In practice, the therapist can never be sure whether information thought to be introduced for the first time is, in fact, new. However, whether or not the information is completely new to the client may not matter to the progress of information processing. The client's reaction will provide the necessary clues as to how much explanation is needed to get the information sufficiently recorded, and/or accessed, to allow for integration as the work continues.

therapist may suggest and lead a relaxation exercise to block the further accessing of anxiety.

I propose that these four categories of EMDR activity, namely,

1. Accessing existing information
2. Introducing new information
3. Facilitating information processing
4. Inhibiting accessing of information

encompass the therapeutic activity of all methods of treatment; this four-activity model (FAM) is a useful guide for organizing thinking about therapeutic interventions.

Category 1. Accessing Existing Information

This activity involves bringing already stored information to, or near, aware-ness. It may include all aspects of past events, such as pictorial representa-tions, thoughts, odors, emotions, sensations, and motor responses. Some of this information is accessed from declarative memory systems, such as the date of an event, or the fact that the event is in the past, or that something positive was learned from it. Other information, such as conditioned emo-tional responses, is accessed from nondeclarative systems. Information accessed will not always be memory of a real event; it may be in the form of a principle or goal, or it may even pertain to an imagined event. In other words, wherever or however information is held, accessing is bringing up what is already there.

All therapeutic relationships begin with an accessing component. When the client initiates phone contact and the therapist first responds, information is accessed immediately. (Analysts would call this the beginning of the transference.) Differences among accessed material can easily be seen if one notes what associations might come to a veteran walking into a government medical center vs. one entering the luxurious office of a practitioner located in a prosperous area.

Different methods of psychotherapy focus on one or another aspect of the information networks. The aspect(s) of networks focused on, and the emphasis on the *way* in which networks are accessed, are a large part of what distinguishes one method from another. For example, psychodynamic therapies traditionally access information by interpretive questioning and free association. Behavior therapies have different emphasis; for example, systematic desensitization accesses by constructing and using items from stimulus hierarchies, and flooding does so by intensely describing stimuli and responses associated with the target activity or event. Cognitive thera-pies emphasize direct questioning and disputation.

As to aspects of network focus, psychodynamic therapies focus on past events and relationships; interpersonal psychotherapy focuses on current relationships; direct therapeutic exposure methods, such as implosion and flooding, focus on responses to past situations; cognitive therapies such as rational emotive behavior therapy (REBT) focus on extreme beliefs about the self; existential therapies may focus on creation of meaning.

Today, in the United States, most methods cannot be as clearly differentiated by their ultimate goals. Several years ago the line separating the various schools of therapy could easily be drawn, with behaviorists attempting to help clients meet specific behavioral goals, dynamic therapists striving for insight and integration, and humanists hoping for self-actualization. Today, the goals appear to converge around the elimination of DSM IV–defined symptoms. Less cynically, we can see the seeds of convergence of goals in Freud's early proclamation that the goal of therapy was to be able to love and to work.

One possible reason EMDR is so quickly and powerfully effective may be the fact that it carefully accesses many aspects of experience. Just prior to the initiation of EM, clients are asked to access visual images, cognitions, emotions, and physical sensations. Much of the clinical section of this book will be about the specifics of accessing information when processing does not go smoothly to resolution. Specifically, knowledge gained from the accessing methods of the rich tradition of psychotherapy will be integrated into EMDR treatment.

Category 2. Introducing New Information

This activity involves the presentation of new information by the therapist, or the encouragement to engage in activity in which information might be acquired.

There are two occasions in therapy when new information is most likely to be explicitly introduced: first, in the explanation of treatment and the formation of treatment plans; and second, when the client lacks the information necessary to add to an unnecessarily painful associative network and thereby achieve adaptive reprocessing.

In all methods of therapy, therapists explicitly provide new information about the treatment they offer. Traditional psychodynamically oriented therapists may introduce information about the unconscious. In an initial discussion, a psychodynamic therapist might explain how early childhood experiences result in conflicts that occur outside awareness, and that these conflicts might then lead to the mysterious presence of anxiety. Behavior therapists introduce information about reinforcement. In an initial discussion, a behavior therapist might explain how being punished in certain situations could lead to an anxiety response in similar later situations, even if a person wasn't aware of the similarities.

In addition to information about the therapy itself, therapists also explicitly introduce new information during the course of treatment. Many methods of therapy focus on the teaching of new information. Behavioral and socially oriented therapies may have clients engage in roleplaying or activity outside the therapist's office that exposes the client to new situations and calls for new responses. In all methods of therapy, the therapist occasionally presents normative data; for example, when during conversation it becomes clear the client doesn't realize that everyone experiences fear in combat or that perpetrators of abuse manipulate their victims into feeling responsible for the abuse.

It may also be that implicitly provided new information, common to all forms of therapy, creates or further develops associations that lead to positive processing. Sometimes just the introduction of explanatory information allows some relief; clients feel better when they hear that their problems have explanations. In some cases, the belief "I am hopelessly, inexplicably, and permanently defective" — which is part of the problem associative network — has a chance to be replaced by, or at least accompanied by, a belief such as, "My problems can be understood and I might be able to feel better." Even more fundamentally, it may be a new insight for the client to learn that a person in a position of authority, such as the therapist, can treat him in a friendly, helpful, noncontrolling manner.

These two pieces of information — that problems can be explained and that someone in authority can be an ally — may be the most powerful information the therapist can impart. This may account for such similar results from different schools of therapy, outside of work with highly specific behaviorally defined problems — as well as positive results from nontherapists (see review by Lambert 1992). Some of the new information emphasized by EMDR that is unique in its combination includes: (1) the client may respond quickly; (2) there is a possible positive cognition, which is explicitly stated; and (3) whatever thoughts come to the client during the course of treatment are acceptable and part of the treatment.

Category 3. Facilitating Information Processing

The impetus to add this category comes from Shapiro's early efforts to describe what to do when a client appears to be "stuck"; that is, if the content of awareness did not change as EMDR progressed. Shapiro's first suggestion was to change the direction of the EM; she then suggested accessing from among visual, auditory, conceptual, and other aspects of the target associative networks in various ways. These various methods of accessing borrowed, as mentioned earlier, from the variety of existing psychotherapy methods. All of the things that could be done (Socratic questioning, two-chair technique, focusing on different aspects of a target picture) preceding eye movement at this especially creative time in treatment (when processing was stuck) seemed to be a different class of activity than the EM. All had a specific type of content — whether an emotion, visual image, or thought — they were trying to elicit, the goal being to integrate that content with other elements. In contrast, the EM, while it may access something, was primarily initiated to integrate.

So, in order to define category activity in a more general way than just saying it is EM, I propose that Category 3 consists of abstract activities whose main purpose is to accelerate, or make more efficient, the integration of accessed or introduced elements. Of the four types of activity proposed, this category is novel and the most difficult to explain. One source of difficulty is the fact that the overt activities have only recently been suggested as being psychotherapeutically successful, and little is known about how they convey their effects. It is also difficult because, in a sense, all therapeutic activities have the goal of facilitating information processing — thus, the name of the category may lead to some confusion, as my colleague William Zangwill (1997, personal communication) has pointed out. Perhaps it will be helpful to consider that previous methods relied on the covert, natural processing the mind does when there is no overt accelerator such as EM.

It may be helpful to distinguish information processing from the other things that can happen to information: acquisition, storage, and retrieval. Successful human information processing is the active communication, or sharing, among associative networks, which usually results in an adaptive transformation of the information. The lack of information processing (that is, the failure of associative networks to intercommunicate), results in limitations on adaptive transformation. Clinically, the extensive failure of networks to communicate is sometimes called dissociation.

To clarify: when a traumatic event is remembered as if it is still happening, and is always interpreted substantially in the same way, from only one point of view, as it was first experienced, then that event is acquired, stored, and retrieved, but only minimally processed. (It is probably stored, and somewhat isolated, in nondeclarative memory systems.[3]) When that same event is remembered as occurring in the past and can be perceived and accepted in many different ways (including being viewed from different visual perspectives), and is not accompanied by excessive emotion or the blocking of emotion, then it is processed.

There are different degrees of processing. Suppose a person is traumatized in a fire and does not process the event. If she sees a fire in a movie, she may have a dissociative experience, acting as if she were reliving the event; alternatively, she may block out almost all emotion. If, instead, she partially processes the event, in the same situation she may simply exhibit excessive levels of fear. Partial processing of a traumatic event may also result in the resolution of emotional distress about the event, without any gain in understanding from the experience.

Complete processing includes not only elimination of the excessive negative emotion, but also fosters some positive resolution, such as recognition of strength in surviving, or the determination to take adaptive (non-compulsively neurotic) steps to avoid such situations in the future. For a person who acted in a regrettable way, perhaps this might mean gratitude for the chance to do better in the future. Complete processing might even include a positive shift in self or world view schema, such as a change from considering oneself

---

3. These memory systems include chiefly nonverbal learned material, such as conditional responses, habituation, complex motor patterns (Squire 1986).

a victim to recognizing that knowledge gained can be shared with others, thus seeing oneself as a teacher.[4]

Activities involved in Category 3 are abstract; they do not in themselves convey information. They are not inherently strongly pleasant or aversive. (This is in contrast to something like a relaxation response, abstract in that it contains no semantic information, but inherently comfortable.) While painful material is being processed and, in being processed, leads one to access more painful material, the experience of the Category 3 activity will be painful. As resolution comes and positive material is processed, positive feelings will accompany Category 3 activities. It is recognized that as a byproduct of processing, accessing will also occur; however, accessing is not the essential aim of Category 3 activities. It is perfectly satisfactory if there is no new evident accessing within the target associative network, so long as it is not needed for integration of associative networks and resolution of a problem.

Few methods of therapy employ overt Category 3 activity. EMDR does with its eye movement and other repetitive sensory/motor activities. A method of treatment called Thought Field Therapy (TFT) may also use a Category 3 activity. In the primary treatment phase, TFT involves having the client (1) simply be aware of a target fear, a traumatic event, or even an urge to engage in an addictive behavior; (2) rate the strength of the accompanying emotion; and then (3) engage in a series of self-tapping, or other simple, self-generated, sensory, motor and/or verbal behaviors (counting or humming) specifically designed for the nature of the problem. Roger Callahan (1995), the originator of the method, reports that his diagnostic procedures are based on applied kinesiology, and that sites selected for stimulation are based on acupuncture points. As of this writing, there is limited independent support from an open therapeutic trial for the effectiveness of TFT in desensitization (Figley and Carbonell 1995), but none for Callahan's proposed mechanism of change.

The Counting Method developed by Frank Ochenberg (1996), in which the therapist counts out loud from 1 to 100 while the client recalls a target traumatic episode, is another method that may employ Category 3 activity. Ochenberg has reported successful results in case studies in less time than is usually afforded learning-theory-based exposure methods. More scientific investigation on this method is being conducted.

I will describe some of the proposed Category 3 activities in more detail. The EM procedure Shapiro introduced in her first articles consisted of the client moving his or her eyes, following the therapist's hand across the length of the client's horizontal field of vision for approximately 24 back-and-forth sweeps, one per second. If the client reported a headache, the therapist

---

4. The reconceptualization of a person who has been traumatically injured from victim to survivor to witness has gained popular currency. I think the next step is that of teacher, whether a formal role or just to people one has ordinary contact with. Each of these steps means giving up something. This will be elaborated on later, in sections on treatment and impediments to therapeutic progress.

alternated to a diagonal motion. Gradually all manner of directions, including circles and infinity symbols, were incorporated by clinicians.

The length of EM also varied. As the method evolved, therapists were instructed to continue EM if the client was showing strong emotional reaction, until distress subsided. Some clinicians report that clients benefited from processing protracted episodes of torture or abuse in sets of 10 or 20 minutes or longer. Clinically, it was observed that clients who began to have difficulty following the therapist's fingers, or who spontaneously stopped moving their eyes, tended to dissociate at those times. Therefore, therapists were instructed to actively verbally encourage clients to resume EM if they stopped.

As early as 1991 (but still *after* naming the method for eye movement) Shapiro, following up on suggestions of EMDR therapists such as Robbie Dunton, was also teaching therapists to use alternative stimulation. She had therapists snap their fingers near one ear and then the other, alternately and repetitively. Similarly, the therapist sometimes used tactile stimulation, having the client rest his palms on his knees while the therapist alternately tapped the palms. Some therapists later reported that having clients — especially those who were very sensitive to physical contact (and had strong dissociative responses) — tap their own knees, worked well; others have children, especially, hit the therapist's palms in a "patty cake" manner.

It may be that not all Category 3 activities have the same type of information processing effect. It is possible that they vary in intensity of effect, type of information most influenced, or a variety of other ways. The effect of Category 3 activity would also undoubtedly be affected by the context. More thorough information processing would be expected if accessing activity is more inclusive, as in standard EMDR, and less thorough if less inclusive. In its extreme, overwhelming dissociation producing accessing in which the client stops participating in the Category 3 activity would not have this positive effect.

More conventional methods of treatment do not add an overt abstract activity, such as eye movement, but rather facilitate processing through timing, repetition, or through the manner in which they access existing information or introduce new information. For example, in systematic desensitization the accessing of less traumatic images occurs before accessing of more traumatic images, which its practitioners believe leads to a greater likelihood of processing than the reverse order. Also in systematic desensitization, the relaxation is accessed in temporal proximity accessing of fear. With flooding, the facilitative abstract activity would be the frequency of accessing the target associative network. In psychodynamic therapy, the therapist carefully times the moment at which he or she reminds the client of a past emotional overreaction so as to (in information processing terms) foster adaptive reprocessing.

Nonsemantic activity that does occur in more traditional treatments — for example, the use of various aversive measures found in some forms of behavior therapy — would not be considered Category 3 activity because it conveys meaning that it is hoped will be connected to target material.

In some situations the introduction of aversive activity would chiefly be a Category 1 activity: the client is reminded of a past discomfort, already in an associative network, that it is hoped will connect more powerfully to a particular behavior or thought. In some circumstances the presentation of an aversive stimulus would be used as a Category 4 activity (described later), to inhibit accessing of an associative network, specifically the behavior that is targeted for suppression.

Orienting Response

It is beyond the scope of this work to extensively explore possible mechanisms by which Category 3 activity may have its effects; however, one possibility is through the orienting response. In discussions of a possible mechanism for EMDR effects with a colleague, Jim Moore, the concept of an "alertness response" was raised. I soon switched to thinking of this by its standard name, the "orienting response" (Lipke 1992). Nat Denny later independently made a similar suggestion and elaborated on it in a paper in *Traumatology* (1995). Armstrong and Vaughn (1996) have independently further elaborated this model and compared it to a classical conditioning explanation of EMDR effects. Denny, in summarizing previous work on the orienting response (OR), noted that psychophysiology investigators starting with Pavlov have developed the idea that some stimuli can interfere with a conditioned response. If what has blocked processing has been a conditioned emotional response such as fear or anger, then partial suppression of this response with Category 3 activity would permit processing to continue. The OR hypothesis is also attractive in that it would allow habituation to explain why changing the direction of EM sometimes results in continuation of processing that appeared to be blocked.

It might be argued that Category 3 activity, in that it is suppressing negative emotion, is inherently experienced as positive, and therefore belongs in Category 4. I am arguing, based on the empirical evidence cited, that if it is inhibition, there are different kinds of inhibition; some, such as EM, promote integration of associative networks, some promote integration. I am also arguing that the effect of inhibitory activity that suppresses the experience of an associative network is different from an inhibitory activity, such as EM, that may lead to the more thorough experience of that network. If EM and other Category 3 activities are to be considered inhibitory, then I would be proposing two categories of inhibitory therapeutic activity, with Category 3 referred to facilitative inhibition.

I also believe that the overall evidence is inconsistent with the counter-conditioning idea of pairing distressing material with relaxation response, or a general decreased activation.

Empirical Evidence on Category 3

Now that Category 3 has been described in general terms, at least roughly, and a possible mechanism of action has been proposed, the obligation arises to more formally justify its existence and to distinguish it from other activities. The initial justification for this category of activities comes from the necessity to explain Shapiro's initial results and the clinical observations reported by many clinicians, including my own. These include:

1. Some cases of desensitization and integration that took place in just a few minutes, to stimuli that had provoked extreme emotional reactions for years and had sometimes been intractable to many interventions.

McCann describes the case of a 41-year-old welder in a mining accident in 1983. He lost both his arms and became completely deaf secondary to antibiotic treatment. Leg injuries required special shoes to enable walking and he had numerous other scars. He had gained some self-sufficiency with sophisticated equipment, and had become a skilled lip reader. He reported that he daily experienced nightmares and flashbacks. "He would see himself being consumed by fire and feel himself gasping for air" (p. 320). He had even more severe anniversary reactions. He avoided television to avoid news stories of fires. He reported frequent insomnia, difficulty concentrating, and startle responses. He reported he had no psychiatric difficulties prior to the accident. In 1991, after two sessions for evaluation, he completed one session of EMD. During this session he processed three separate scenes from this accident and one from an earlier accident. He did one set of eye movements with each scene, each time spontaneously reporting that a new scene came to mind: the next scene was of him peacefully floating on a cloud, accompanied by the words "I'm alive."

When he returned a week later, he reported feeling "really good." Among other positive reactions, he said he now placed himself in the "can do category." His nurse described him as "happier" and more responsible for himself, managing entirely on his own for hours at a time. He had not been on his own since the accident. One month later, his rehabilitation counselor reported that the subject had passed his driving course and was now driving himself around town. When asked to comment on the EMD, the subject said "It was a relief. A boulder was lifted off me."

Other changes attributed to the EMD were the ability to watch television scenes with fires and not have flashbacks, resolution of anxiety, and passing the anniversary date with continued improvement. This is the most dramatic of several reports by therapists of brief effective treatment of severe problems (Cocco and Sharpe 1993; Kleinknecht 1993; Shapiro 1989b; Spates and Burnette 1995).

2. Incidents I have observed in which these rapid changes are reported by the client, or are experienced by the therapist in his or her own use of EMDR, to have occurred during the EM. My first such observation is reported in Lipke and Botkin (1993); a client who, in 15 minutes, found resolution with an incident he had failed to make gains with in the previous 3 months of inpatient treatment.

3. The commonly made clinical observation that, for the same client, eye movement will accompany intense emotion, both negative and positive. Often clients begin a set of eye movements in a moderately negative affective state; as the set of eye movements progress, clients move through intense negative emotion, such as fear or panic, then by the end of the set become calm or even euphoric. Among the most startling examples are clients who process the trauma of near-drowning: as eye movement progresses, the clients are panicked and choking, then move toward the calmness that goes with resolution.

4. Clients stated a preference for eye movement or other Category 3 activity, as compared to no activity (Boudewyns and Hyer 1996). Based on clinical results that far exceeded anything my clients had been able to achieve prior to EMDR, and on frequent client requests for Category 3 activity, I had not varied from standard Category 3 activity. Recently, after some scientists (see extensive review below) reported that, based on their data, they believed what I call the Category 3 activity was unnecessary, I asked some clients who had been treated in numerous conventional EMDR sessions to either close their eyes or stare straight ahead during the time I would have normally asked them to participate in Category 3 activity. I then asked each if they preferred the EM (or other usual activity) or the less active one they had just completed. All clients preferred the Category 3 activity and, consistent with the observation that the activity does not have consistent immediate hedonic or aversive effects, some preferred it because they found it more relaxing and some because it stirred things up more. (Of course, these testimonials do not constitute proof; they do, however, provide clues.)

In addition to the clinical observations of change occurring immediately following EM, results of EMDR have been attributed to the EM (and later, as other results became available, to other Category 3 activity) because of the absence of traditional theoretical explanation to account for the clinical observations. There are too many violations of standard exposure therapy rules (brief and interrupted exposure,[5] encouragement of free association, rather than attendance to target stimuli) and too many incidents of rapid therapeutic response for the method to be explained by conventional learning theories (for example, extinction, counterconditioning). As to cognitive behavioral explanations, the cognitive component in many successful EMDR cases, such as McCann's, is too weak to carry this load. Also relevant is the timing of observed client change: it is observed after eye movement, not after the establishment of the negative and positive cognitions. I have observed this to be true even when the cognitive component is introduced, as I do in the session before Category 3 activity begins. In addition, there is

5. Rodriguez and Craske (1993), reviewing the literature on exposure treatment of phobia state: "All of the theories which state the possible role of distraction during fear reduction suggest a negative impact" (p. 550).

no record of systematically observed rapid cognitive therapy success with chronic severe PTSD.

Similarly, psychodynamic explanations do not have empirical support for rapidly effective results. Psychodynamic theory would generally predict that such rapid responses would be temporary, or result in symptom substitution, neither of which has been found in the follow-up data on EMDR treatment, as noted in studies reviewed in Chapter 1.

Category 3 activity may turn out not to be viable, but it is difficult to imagine what explanation of the above-described clinical findings might be invoked that does not involve eye movement, tapping, or an alternative activity. However, if an exposure explanation is finally supported, then perhaps Shapiro will be credited with inadvertently demonstrating that imaginal exposure can be accomplished a lot more effectively and painlessly if done in the way she prescribes. This in itself would be a major breakthrough, given the failure of imaginal exposure, a scientifically validated treatment method, to be extensively used to treat the effects of psychological trauma.[6]

Although the clinical observations of EMDR treatment are unique and surprising, and the logic of attributing these results to Category 3 activity is compelling, from a treatment planning point of view it would be impossible to abandon EM or other Category 3 activity given the reports of my clients. However, scientific acceptance of the importance of Category 3 activity will rest on controlled scientific studies.

Researchers have attempted to assess the role of EM, hand tapping, and auditory stimulation in EMDR in a number of studies. This body of literature, though small, is quite messy. Although I will start by reviewing studies that consider the role of EM in EMDR, that is not the primary purpose of this review; rather, it is to consider some general questions regarding the definition of Category 3 activity and its effects. Empirically, defining Category 3 presents the problems of circularity and aiming at a moving target.

To work our way out of this morass, we begin by defining Category 3 activities as EM, hand tapping, and alternate auditory stimulation. These are activities that have been part of EMDR treatments, and have been observed to be part of clinically effective treatment. Note, again, that Category 3 does not include activities that are strongly aversive in themselves, such as painful shocks; Category 3 activities are intended to carry information, in the hope that it will connect with target associative networks.

The next step is to demonstrate that proposed Category 3 activities add something to the therapeutic process. If and when this is established, then

6. This conclusion is based on my personal observation of practicing clinicians and is supported by a survey I conducted of inpatient PTSD treatment programs designed for intensive trauma work with combat veterans in the DVA medical system. During the period of this survey, I was able to contact the directors of 17 of the 21 programs. Six programs, for a total of 18 clinicians, were reported to be using exposure methods as reported on by Keane, Boudewyns, and other researchers. Thirteen programs, with a total of 32 clinicians, were using EMDR.

the goal of research will be to isolate the activities and understand the mechanism of effect.

To recap, I initially defined activities in this category by their inclusion in EMDR, by their phenomenological uniqueness, and by association with unusually powerful treatment effects. I will next explore the experimental data, first concerning the clinical value of EM, and then concerning the category's other proposed activities. The final step will then be to briefly consider the mechanism of effect, as this last step is largely beyond the scope of this book.

Review of the Studies

It is reasonable to propose that when a new "fact" is discovered the burden of proof, through replicated experimental demonstration, is on the discoverer. At some point, however, after the effect has been demonstrated repeatedly, failure to replicate can be taken as demonstration of the limitations of the failed replications, or limitations of the robustness of the proposed effect, rather than negation of the effect.

At this writing, there are several studies that may be interpreted as providing at least some support for the notion that eye movement in itself, or in an EMDR context, may promote processing. Two of these focus on only the effect of EMDR-like eye movement in nonclinical situations.

Andrade, Kavanagh, and Baddeley (1997), after reviewing literature that suggests eye movement decreases the intensity of visual imagery in general, and disrupts memory dependent on visual cues, studied the effects of EMDR-like eye movement on image intensity and emotion associated with images. In this nonclinical controlled study, EMDR-like lateral eye movement resulted in less imagic vividness, as well as less emotional reaction to both positive and negative imagery, when compared to both a no-eye-movement and a simple spatial pattern tapping condition. Complex spatial pattern tapping did, however, lead to less emotional reaction than a simple pattern, or a no-activity control condition.[7]

In the second nonclinical examination of what the authors considered EMDR, Hekmat and his associates (Hekmat, Groth, and Rogers 1994) measured the effects of EMDR, EM with music, and a no-treatment control on pain responses in 30 subjects randomly divided into three groups. Pain tolerance was significantly improved for the two eye-movement groups, compared to the notreatment control. All subjects were given the Harvard Hypnotic Susceptibility Scale as a pretest. EM subjects were divided into two subgroups; one group in each condition did lateral EM and one group in each condition did movements in an infinity sign pattern. The results showed that statistically both EM treatments were significantly superior to the control condition in pain threshold, tolerance, and endurance. The infinity figure movement

---

7. Ironically, Andrade et al., buying into a Herbert and Meuser critique, conclude that EMDR itself may not be effective psychotherapy, but suggest that the eye movement component be salvaged as potentially contributing to some other kind of effective psychotherapeutic procedure.

seemed to have a slight advantage for the music group. Hypnotizability had no influence.

This study certainly cannot be considered definitive; however, it does support the effects of EM and also suggests that EM effects are different from hypnosis effects.

The remainder of the studies that appear to lend some support to the effects of Category 3 activity focus on clinical problems.

Gosselin and Matthews (1995), in studying test anxiety, compared standard EMDR with EMDR protocol, but substituted staring at the therapist's unmoving fingers for EM. They found that, while all subjects improved, EM produced significantly more SUD improvement than no EM. This study controlled for expectancy, and found no difference between groups on this variable. Both groups appeared to benefit similarly on the Test Anxiety Inventory, administered 1 month posttreatment.

Feske and Goldstein (1997) studied EMDR with panic attacks, comparing five sessions of EMDR to a waitlist control group. They then compared EMDR to EMDR with subjects' eyes fixed (EF) on the therapist's finger substituted for EM. The therapists in this study were trained in EMDR and also had some of their sessions positively reviewed for treatment fidelity by an EMDR teacher. Subjects showed statistically and clinically significant improvement, and superiority to the waitlist group on the standard measures used. More relevant to the Category 3 question, the EM group showed significantly more improvement on two of five measures. However, at 3-month follow-up, the groups were equivalent.

Prior to the above-mentioned listed study by Boudewyns, he and some of the same research team cited above conducted a pilot study in a Veterans Administration treatment program for chronic combat-related PTSD (Boudewyns et al. 1990). After several subjects dropped for various reasons, nine subjects were treated with two sessions of EMDR, six with a variant that eliminated EM (the details of this were not reported), and five were in a no-treatment control group. Not surprisingly for this population, none of the groups showed significant pre to post improvement on the standard measures used. However, the EM group did report significant decreases in SUDs scores related to the target trauma.

Surprisingly, strong support for the importance of EM in EMDR has come from the most virulent critics of the method, Lohr, Tolin, and Montgomery (1995). Lohr and Tolin, with Kleinknecht (1995, 1996), published two papers with two case studies each. In these studies, they applied a variant of the EMDR protocol, first without EM and then with EM. Subjects consistently reported no significant decrease in distress until the EM were added. For the blood and medical procedures, phobia subjects who received the dismantling procedure, Lohr, Tolin, and Kleinknecht (1995) concluded that the subject:

> Both subjects' verbal reports of fear changed substan-
> tially when eye movements were added to the general
> protocol. It was concluded that the addition of eye

> movements was necessary to reduce the aversiveness
> of some phobic imagery. (p. 73)

Similar findings were reported for two medical phobic subjects treated in the 1996 study.

Concurrent measures of heart rate were also used: these failed to show significant changes throughout the treatment, even when subjective reports indicated decreased anxiety. While failure to show heart rate decreases diminishes the strength of the argument, it does not undermine it. It may be noted that emotion is highly complexly experienced, physiological baselines differ from person to person, and physiological measures in themselves do not speak unequivocally. Elevated heart rate is associated with happiness as well as fear (Ekman, Levenson, and Freisen 1983). Thus, given the subjects' report of alleviation of anxiety, we may speculate that along with small residual fear, subjects were experiencing happiness that the fear was decreasing. This could account for the lack of statistical significance in change in physiology. This hypothesis is especially consistent with EMDR, since it is designed to be not just a desensitization procedure, but one that includes positive reprocessing.

Montgomery and Ayllon (1994), using a multiple baseline design, attempted to measure the contribution of EM to the EMDR procedure in the treatment of non-combat-related PTSD. Montgomery and Ayllon subjects participated in four conditions in a fixed order, but with random variation in number of sessions:

1. Baseline measures, 3 to 5 sessions
2. An approximation of EMDR, with staring at a point substituted for EM (EF condition), 3 to 5 sessions
3. An approximation of EMDR, 6 sessions
4. Follow-up, 2 to 6 sessions

The authors reported statistically significant and substantial clinical gains for their subjects. These improvements were recorded on SUD and behavioral measures, including intrusive thoughts and dreams. No significant gains or trends were attributed to the non-EM condition; the observed improvement was attributed to the EM condition. Heart rate drops appeared attributable to the EM condition, but failed to reach significance for the group, possibly because two of the six subjects started with heart rates close to normal resting rate. (Heart rate may also have been lower because this measure was taken across many sessions and the "happiness effect" may have worn off.)

Unfortunately, it appears that the therapists in this study were not authoritatively trained in the method and varied their instructions and timing, which limits the generalizability of their results. Nevertheless, these results may be added to evidence, from at least one EMDR critic, supporting EM as facilitating treatment effects.

A Renfrey and Spates (1994) study, at first glance, appears not to support the effect of EM as an active ingredient in treatment. In treating severely traumatized subjects, most of whom met stringent criteria for PTSD, they compared three conditions: (1) standard EMDR; (2) EMDR using a blinking light instead of a moving hand to lead EM; and (3) focusing on a fixed light as a substitute for rapid eye movements. When discussing the effectiveness of EMDR, subjects in all three groups reported clinically and statistically impressive improvement. Two features of the study suggest support for the Category 3 hypothesis, despite the similar results in all three groups on most measures. First, the nature of the no-EM task, encouraged focus on a point, so that subjects may have been engaging in Category 3 activity. The apparent non-EM group did engage in some EM: when the therapist noted that subjects' eyes stopped converging on the light, the light blinked until it was again focused on; if that did not work, the therapist provided a verbal prompt.

Also, sustained focus on a point may itself be a Category 3 activity. Mulholland and Peper (1971) have demonstrated that ocular convergence produces a shift to alpha wave production. The relevance of this observation may be enhanced when one considers that a shift to dissociation is often accompanied by a nonconvergent "blank stare." However, its importance is undermined by the number of studies that show EM to be more effective than staring at a point (Lohr et al. 1995, 1996; Andrade et al. 1997).

Statistically non-significant but substantial differences in treatment time to achieve desensitization may also be telling. The two EM groups achieved criterion in a mean of 3.9 and 4.3 sessions, engaging in 43.5 and 40.3 sets of EM. Subjects who stare at a light averaged 5.4 sessions to reach criterion and 57.6 sets of visual attention. When Renfrey and Spates looked at PTSD diagnosis for the two EM groups, 13 of the 15 subjects who met criteria for DSM-IIIR diagnosis of PTSD prior to treatment no longer met criteria on 3-month follow-up, whereas in the eye-fixation group, only 3 of 6 subjects who had met this criteria no longer did so. Though statistical comparisons reported by Renfrey and Spates do not show significant differences between the groups, the finding that 13 of 15 subjects no longer fall into the PTSD group is impressively high.

Studies Unsupportive of Category 3

The first study considered suggests that to isolate the effect of EM, one must be careful that the problem studied is difficult enough so that rapid results are not achieved simply by means of the non-Category-3 activity used in EMDR, or in other treatment methods. Foley and Spates (1995), in treating college students with fear of public speaking, compared standard EMDR to EMDR substituting (1) alternating auditory stimulation, or (2) clients looking at their hands, for EM. They also included a no-treatment control group. They found significant positive effects with all three variations, and concluded that EMDR was effective, but that with the population studied EM were not essential to treatment. This statement could have been made more strongly if there had been authoritative monitoring of the EMDR treatment.

However, the central point here is that, since EMDR has components that are parts of already established methods of psychotherapy, any added value of Category 3 activity may not be evident in some tests.

Foley and Spates also suggest that the results of all three groups are equivalent because the operative factor that EMDR brings to treatment is dosed flooding. While this may be an important factor in EMDR, support of this hypothesis contradicts the widely accepted theory, noted previously, that longer exposure periods are more effective than shorter ones (experimentally supported by Stern and Marks 1972; Grayson et al. 1982; and summarized by Rodriguez and Craske 1993), and that for exposure to be most effective it has to continue until there is a decrease in distress.

In another study, Sanderson and Carpenter (1992) attempted to evaluate the role of EM in EMDR, but had methodological problems that undercut their finding that EMDR-type eye movements were inconsequential in EMDR-type therapy. They treated a variety of phobic subjects in a crossover design, using both what they thought was EMD and a similar procedure in which subjects closed their eyes instead of doing EM. They found similar positive results with both groups. Unfortunately, there were several violations of standard EMDR instructions and protocol, including apparent failure to make client-produced associations the target of each new set of eye movements.

The Sanderson and Carpenter finding that some positive effects are shown may imply that interrupted exposure has some positive effects, and/or it may imply that their instructions to maintain discomfort overwhelm Category 3 effects, but their results cannot be evidence on the question of the existence of the category. It should also be noted that a similar lack of differentiation between EM and a no-EM condition was obtained by Acierno et al. (1994) in one multiply phobic subject, also mistakenly instructed to retain the target image, thoughts, and sensation throughout the EM phase. It also appears that neither the Sanderson and Carpenter (1992) study nor the Acierno et al. (1994) study used independent assessment of results.

Boudewyns and Hyer (1996), as mentioned previously, studied subjects who already received continuing standard care for combat-related PTSD. For these subjects, the attempt was to compare conventional EMDR with a variant in which subjects closed their eyes instead of engaging in EM; a third group who received only standard care was included. The subjects receiving EMDR and the variant both improved significantly on a number of measures, including psychophysiological response to trauma stimuli. There was no difference between the two groups on the standard measures, though clients and therapists preferred the EM to the no-EM condition. The flaws in this study were primarily the failure of the design to allow enough time within each session to work through trauma and to have clients engage in stress-reduction exercises for sessions in which processing was incomplete.[8] These

8. As with the Pitman et al. (1996) study, tapes of the EMDR sessions were observed by the author as a consultant to this study. As a consultant, I must bear some responsibility for the study's problems.

problems, as well as the tendency of therapists to lead rather than follow clients, may have led to limiting results of the therapeutic response, thereby making it difficult to reach conclusions about the role of the Category 3 activity in the EMDR protocol.

In a yoked control design, Dunn and associates (1996) attempted to assess the role of EM in EMDR with college students recruited to participate in a study; the students were told that researchers were examining a method to help reduce stress in people who were emotionally traumatized. Twenty-eight subjects participated. Subjects in the non-EM condition, which the authors referred to as placebo, stared at a dot on a piece of paper 1 to 3 feet away. Both the EM and "placebo" groups showed some improvement on several psychophysiology measures. While the mean SUD decrease in the EM group was greater than that of the "placebo" group (3.3 vs. 2.4), the difference between groups was not statistically significant.

The relevance of this study on the Category 3 questions may be diminished by the fact that Dunn et al. limited therapy sessions to 45 minutes, violating the principle that there must be allowance for initial increases in distress, and sufficient time for therapeutic effects to be accomplished — especially in a first session. Ironically, the authors cite the time constriction as an advantage of the EM condition. In evaluating the usefulness of this study in informing the decision about the viability of Category 3, it is important to consider that Category 3 activity is postulated to be effective with clinically relevant material when applied in a context that would promote processing.

Whether the Dunn group understood that EM or any other intervention, to be successful, must access such a context (or at least *not access* threat context cues that overwhelm possible therapeutic effects) was called into question in the discussion section of the paper. After they completed work with the subjects who were part of the yoked design, they decided to explore "placebo" effects by subjecting additional subjects to the identical treatment.

This time, subjects were told that the EMDR procedures were simply "testing the effects of visual stimuli on stressful or traumatic experiences." They reported that all three pairs of subjects reported feeling worse, and three subjects broke into tears. The procedure was stopped then, because the experimenter thought it might be harmful. The authors concluded then that "experimenter/therapist-induced expectations may play a significant role in the use of EMDR procedures." Dunn et al. apparently failed to recognize that expectancy effects influence every social interaction and other methods of psychotherapy. The focus on expectancy effects, rather than on how their application of EMDR, by not preparing the client for a possible negative response, was evidence that they were not using EM in a context that could maximize and demonstrate its effect, or demonstrate its limitations through failure to surpass the convergent focus variant.

In an unpublished doctoral dissertation, Opdyke (1995) offered subjects with PTSD two sessions of either standard EMDR, or a variation of EMDR in which subjects were instructed to continuously stare at a spot on the opposite wall while the therapist encouraged them to maintain their eye focus. The ten subjects in each group showed significant pre to post improvement on two standard measures of PTSD, as well as on SUD scores. There were no statistically significant differences in improvement shown by the two treatment groups — except that the eye-movement group showed significant improvement on the VoC, while the eye focus group did not — although it did show a strong trend toward improvement on that measure. There was no improvement on any measure for the waitlist control group.

Opdyke attributed his positive results to exposure effects or to placebo effects. The exposure explanation was discussed above. The placebo explanation presents its own difficulties, in that Opdyke's "placebo results" would make his placebo more powerful in therapeutic effect in two sessions than "active" therapies have been in many more sessions. One interpretation of Opdyke's findings, as well as the findings of the other studies demonstrating positive effects for the no-eye-movement "placebo" condition, suggests that the maintained convergence on the spot on the wall in front of non-EM subjects, especially when accompanied by the eye movements involved in returning to that spot and the therapist's verbal encouragement to maintain visual focus, were sufficient to meet Category 3 requirements. Some psychophysiological support for eye convergence as similar to EMDR-type EM comes from work by Mulholland and Peper (1971), mentioned briefly above, who report that convergence and some types of eye movement suppress occipital and parito-occipital alpha, whereas a nonconvergent, fixed stare seems to promote alpha. The relevance of this may be enhanced when one considers the clinical observation that a shift to dissociation is often accompanied by a nonconvergent "blank stare." The importance of this observation is tempered by the studies reviewed below that suggest EM is superior to eye fixation as a component of EMDR treatment.

Non-EM Activities

The first study reviewed in this section is judged to support the notion that EM is not unique in facilitating reprocessing, but is rather one of a category of activities that performs this function. Treating chronic combat-related PTSD, Pitman et al. compared standard EMDR with a version that had subjects, instead of moving their eyes, tap their hands on the arms of their chairs, and stare at a mark on the opposite wall while the therapist moved his fingers across their field of vision in the manner of conventional EMDR. The goal of this design was to have comparable psychophysiological activity in both groups.

Subjects in both groups reported "modest to moderate" (p. 419) improvement, especially on the Impact of Events Scale, but no improvement on most global measures. Pitman et al. concluded that EMDR — either the EM or fixed-eyes version — yields results at least comparable to those of standard exposure, but with better acceptability to clients. The Pitman results appear to support the notion of an expanded Category 3. Unfortunately, interpretations of this group's findings must be limited because many of the sessions were often not consistent with the standard practice of EMDR. The most frequent error made by Pitman therapists was failure to follow the subjects' associations and, rather, suggest different foci of attention prior to the subsequent set of Category 3 activity.

It is interesting to note two other findings of the Pitman et al. study. First, there were significant correlations between fidelity to EMDR accessing principles and treatment outcome on several measures, including the CAPS for both groups. Second, three subjects in the EM condition and one subject in the fixed-eyes condition completed desensitization prior to the six sessions allotted.

Devilly, Spence, and Rapee (1998) also treated war veterans with chronic combat-related PTSD. Attempting to study the EM in EMDR, the researchers substituted a variable-rate blinking light, controlled to maintain subject visual attention to it, as a substitute for EM. Although Devilly et al. were disappointed in the magnitude of subject improvement, there were statistically significant improvements for the EMDR and EMDR variation groups over the supportive treatment group on a number of variables. This, despite the fact that only two sessions of treatment were offered to these subjects who had undergone much previous treatment, and still had reported considerable symptomatology at the start of the study. In comparing EM and visual attention groups, there was a consistent, though not statistically different, advantage for the EM group.

A few studies in addition to that of the Pitman group have explicitly looked at what might be considered non-EM Category 3 activity. The study most powerfully supportive of EM is not supportive of alternative activity (the expanded Category 3 hypothesis) was completed by David Wilson and associates (Wilson et al. 1996). Subjects with problems related to traumatic memories received either standard EMDR, EMDR substituting alternate tapping of their own fingers in time to a metronome, or EMDR with a resting period substituted for EM. Subjects in the EM condition reported almost complete relief of subjective distress, as well as significant improvement on SUD and a variety of psychophysiological measures. Subjects in the other two conditions reported and showed almost no improvement until they then received standard EMDR, which resulted in improvement comparable to the standard EMDR group.

The therapists in this study were both highly experienced and competent EMDR practitioners and had assisted Shapiro in the training of other clinicians. This study, while strongly supportive of the effectiveness of EMDR and EM, is not consistent with a Category 3 that would include more than EM. Since clients tapping themselves has been seen to be an effective EM substitute in some clinical situations, the Wilson et al. finding begs for an explanation. Shapiro (1997, personal communication) has suggested that keeping time with a metronome by alternately tapping one's fingers may be too great a distraction and not allow the continued accessing of relevant associative networks. The Wilson study, besides adding complexity to understanding, does prepare the way for the more detailed examination subtleties of what may or may not be a Category 3 activity.

On the other hand, in a study of test anxiety in a nonclinical population, comparing an eye movement version EMDR with a version EMDR substituting subjects' tapping their first fingers on a table in time to a metronome, Bauman and Melnyk (1994) found both treatments to lead to "clinically" and statistically significant improvement on a number of variables. The tapping exercise seemed to lead to slightly more desensitization, while the EM seemed to lead to slightly better processing, as seen in VoC scores.

Finally, in a one-session trial on EMDR, using an auditory variant of the method, Cocco and Sharpe (1993) reported relief of PTSD symptoms in a 4-year-old boy, as monitored by the boy's parents.

What does all this mean for the viability of the EM in EMDR, for alternative activities, and for Category 3? Clearly, the results can only be suggestive because there are too many variables, too few studies, and too much confounding evidence, but here is how I sort it out. The nonclinical study by Andrade et al. (1997) and the clinical studies by Gosselin and Matthews (1995), Montgomery and Ayllon (1994), Lohr et al. (1995, 1996), and D. Wilson et al. (1996) are strongly supportive of EM as relevant. Because of smaller effects or less control on the EM-relevant variables, Feske and Goldstein (1997), Hekmat et al. (1994), Boudewyns et al. (1993) and, I believe, Renfry and Spates (1994) are somewhat supportive. Boudewyns and Hyer (1996), Foley and Spates (1995), Opdyke (1995), Sanderson and Carpenter (1992), Dunn et al. (1996), and Acierno et al. (1994) are nonsupportive or, to varying degrees, contradictory of the effects of EM and the category in general.[9]

The degree to which the negative studies do not support EM may be more suggestive of limitations of the effect rather than absence of effect. Once

---

9. Tallis and Smith (1994) reported a study of "rapid eye movement desensitization" that I find almost impossible to categorize. In a putative effort to understand the role of rapid EM, slower EM, and no EM on desensitization to a photograph of a mutilation, researchers found that instructing subjects to move their closed eyes in time to taps on their shoulders appeared to produce very little change in distress, as opposed to slow tapping (EM) or no EM instructions. This study would be a straightforward argument against EM as a Category 3 activity, except for two considerations: (1) subjects' eyes were closed and there was no evidence reported that clients' closed eyes were actually moving; and, more tellingly, (2) the authors did not employ standard therapist-led EM because a "...pilot conducted by the first author suggested that many patients find it difficult to hold a mental image in mind tracking a finger from side to side." (p. 459) The decision to not use standard EMDR EM in this context may be taken as acknowledgment that EM in standard EMDR is extremely effective. Therefore, contrary to the authors' conclusions, this study may be taken as support of EM as Category 3 activity and not of alternative activity.

This opportunity may be taken to question the biases of Tallis and Smith. In criticizing the dissemination of "REMD" before there is sufficient validation, these authors, after demonstrating anti-EM effect bias in their design, quote me out of context to make it appear that I was making premature, global, and intemperate claims for "REMD." They quote me as saying "...REMD (sic) is 'by far the most effective and efficient treatment' for post traumatic stress disorder." (p. 460) My statement in context was: "EMDR is by far the most effective and efficient treatment we have ever used with dissociative episodes, intrusive memories, and nightmares with Vietnam combat veterans." I was quoted as the former director of PTSD treatment unit. The actual statement, while extremely positive, is limited to effect on specific symptoms, based on clinical observations in a specific environment; of course, now the research supports a stronger stand.

there is a critical mass demonstrating the therapeutic effects of EM, which I believe is present, failures to find the effect are more instructive about the nature of the effect, or the ability of researchers to find it, than they are about the existence of the effect. Psychologists often take the position that if a clinician or researcher produces an effect, everyone must find it in order for it to be established. We may want to consider the possibility that failure to find an effect may be due to poor execution, just as in fields such as medicine or art. Not all surgeons can do every operation, nor can every pianist play a Rachmaninoff piano concerto. Failure in those instances reflects on the performer or performance, not on the activity being performed.

On the question of Category 3 containing activities other than EM, Pitman et al. (1996), Bauman and Melynick (1994), Cocco and Sharpe (1993), Devilly et al. (1998), and Andreade et al. (1997), as well as extensive clinical work, suggest an expanded category. D. Wilson et al. (1996) suggests not. Most of the research suggests an expanded category that would include some variant of bilateral tactile stimulation. Additionally, though it has not been proposed as an EMDR activity, a case could be made for ocular convergence accompanied by therapist prompts and the eye movement necessary to maintain that state as an effective Category 3 activity.

However, if the category is so expanded, I am in danger of being accused of making the argument that anything anyone might do could be construed as Category 3 activity. I suggest, alternatively, that if it is the OR response that provides the mechanism for accelerated information processing with Category 3 activity, then many different activities could produce the kind of sustained OR that leads to the rapid results seen in EMDR, compared to conventional therapies for PTSD.

It is also possible that, for Category 3 activity in general, there is a person by activity by target type interaction that could contribute to an explanation, if there is ever enough research, of the peripatetic findings with both EM and non-EM activities.

Category 4. Inhibition of Information Accessing

Familiar examples of inhibition in psychotherapy are the use of relaxation techniques to decrease anxiety, or turn attention away from troubling images, thoughts, and so forth. Although the most complete purpose of psychotherapy is to process or reprocess information, sometimes an intermediate goal is to help the client isolate information to provide temporary relief of destructive distress. Some form of this activity is used by most psychotherapists. Therapists using EMDR often use inhibition activities to close sessions in which traumatic events are not completely processed. Therapists who employ flooding use relaxation exercises at the end of sessions for similar purpose. Outside the realm of psychotherapy, anxiolytic and neuroleptic medication are commonly used to inhibit the accessing of information.

The inhibitory activity of Category 4 must not be confused with the possible inhibitory effects of Category 3 activity. In the latter, there may be inhibition of some aspect of the conditioned emotional response and/or the avoidance response, which then allows for the processing of information. Inhibition of avoidance, thereby allowing processing, is not the same as the attempt to inhibit accessing of the whole associative network found in Category 4. The essential differences are profound and include purpose, types of activities, and likely outcome.

It also must be recognized that when information is accessed or introduced, whatever was previously in awareness will be inhibited: if you are standing on the corner and see a car, then a bus, the bus can be said to contribute to the inhibition of awareness of the car. Again, the purpose of accessing or introducing new information in psychotherapy is to promote integration, rather than inhibit whatever was in awareness prior to the therapeutic activity. It is as if the therapist drove the car, and then the bus, past the client — not to have the bus take the place of the car in consciousness, but rather to help the client understand that vehicles go past this corner. In Category 4, the therapist asks the driver of the bus to drive in a manner to make it more likely that awareness of the car will be inhibited, and awareness of the bus will be promoted.

The Four-Activity Model in EMDR and Other Methods

With the basics of the FAM model described, it may be useful to more specifically integrate EMDR, other methods of psychotherapy, and the four-activity model. The eight phases of EMDR have *rapport, history taking,* and *contracting components* that share characteristics with other methods, but also have distinctive qualities in EMDR. These early stages of treatment chiefly involve Category 1 activity, accessing existing information networks, and Category 2 activity, introduction of new information. While therapeutic change often occurs when treatment begins, and EMDR can be distinguished from other methods at these stages, the most notable differences begin later in the Assessment and Desensitization phases, where dysfunctional thoughts and emotions are addressed and where the bulk of therapeutic change is expected.

In the Assessment phase, which begins with Category 1 activity, the accessing of stored information, EMDR borrows from — and shares — activities from other treatment methods, but arranges them in a unique way. When this stage begins in EMDR:

1. The client is asked to picture the worst moment of the target event. This is similar to imaginal exposure, but also to any form of therapy in which the therapist asks the client to describe the problem situation. (The examples of similarities between EMDR and other methods are meant to be illustrative, not all-inclusive.)

2. A negative cognition, usually in the form of a self-statement, is identified or developed. This is similar to Rational Emotive Behavior Therapy (REBT),

Cognitive Behavior Therapy (CBT), and the paradoxical intervention of Strategic Therapy.

3. An alternative, positive cognition is identified or developed and then rated for veracity. This step, again, shows similarity to REBT/CBT and, in rating the positive cognition, a core principle of behavior therapy is observed. This stage in EMDR often involves Category 2 activity, as clients may not possess information needed to construct a positive cognition.

4. Emotions and physical sensations present as the event is recalled are identified and rated, again sharing features with body therapies, exposure therapies, and general behavioral principles.

5. The client is asked to bring all negative components of the target event to awareness. The similarity to imaginal exposure therapy is clear.

6. At this point, Category 3 activity, facilitation of information processing (usually 10 seconds or so of eye movement), is initiated.

7. After completing the eye movements, the client is asked what comes to awareness without any prompting from the therapist about type of experience. The client is essentially asked for a free association, borrowing from psychoanalytic approaches and the accepting, nonjudgmental attitude of client-centered therapy.

8. Another round of Category 3 activity is then initiated. In the simplest cases, this pattern continues until the target event is desensitized and reprocessed. As noted previously, phase 6, 7, and 8 activity is very different from standard imaginal exposure procedures, in which the client is urged to maintain attention to distress-provoking stimuli for prolonged periods; distraction from target would be discouraged (Grayson, Foa, and Steketee, 1982; Lyon and Keane, 1989; Stern and Marks, 1972). Thus, it is unlikely that simple extinction is the principal change mechanism in EMDR.

When the process of alternating between Category 3 activities and client statement of the content of awareness does not lead to successful information processing, further Category 1 (accessing) and Category 2 (introduction of information) activities are initiated. These can be borrowed from any number of therapeutic approaches, and will be elaborated on extensively in subsequent chapters. But one example could be asking the client to imagine talking to a person involved in the event (borrowing from Gestalt therapy) prior to a new round of Category 3 activity. Alternatively, a grieving client who believes a loved one is in heaven may be asked to imagine where that person is now (borrowing from pastoral counseling, or perhaps reflecting regression in service of the ego) prior to a new round of Category 3 activity. Finally, at the end of a session, if the client is still experiencing some distress,

Category 4 activity, inhibition of information processing, may be initiated in the form of relaxation exercises or hypnosis.

The four-activity model is a broad outline of psychotherapeutic activity that I see as having the potential to integrate psychotherapeutic modalities from an information processing point of view. As this model is further elaborated and explored, it may help shed light on which particular intervention might be most useful at any given moment in the course of psychotherapy. It may also be noted in passing that clinical formulation in this type of therapeutic process minimizes the importance of medical model diagnostic categories and focuses on the more traditional behavioral formulation in which the specifics of the problem are most important.

Comparing the FAM to Other Metatheories

It may be worthwhile to compare the FAM model to two of the most sophisticated integrative models: the transtheoretical model (TtM) of Prochaska and DiClemente (1992), and Lazarus' (1989) Multimodal Model (MM). To begin with TtM, in this model the goal of therapy, simply stated, is to: "...enable the individual to engage in more accurate information processing." (p. 302) This is close to the description I would use for the most ambitious goal of therapy in the FAM. The goal of *all* therapies from the point of view of the FAM is advancement of information processing. Similarly, Freud (1932, 1964), weighing in on this matter, famously stated:

> Its intention (psycho-analysis) is indeed, to strengthen
> the ego ... to widen its field of perception and enlarge
> its organization so that it can appropriate fresh portions of the id. Where id was ego shall be. (p. 80)

The exception to this information processing goal in the FAM is when a client or therapist decides he does not want to risk confronting the painful aspects of that effort, and instead asks for help in limiting information accessing. In its purest form, this limiting is best represented by Category 4 activities, such as relaxation training, self-hypnosis, or meditation. However, a client engaging in Category 4 activity who repeatedly says to himself "I'm OK, I'm OK" to block negative thoughts, can be seen as accessing a positive belief, even though it is just for the purpose of blocking accessing of the negative belief. Clinical experience teaches us that repetition of a competing belief will not do much for the processing of a strong negative associative network; therefore, this strategy would only secondarily be considered an accessing activity.

One important contribution of the TtM is the integration of therapy-based and nontherapy-based change processes. The TtM model describes change as taking place in six stages. The stages are precontemplation, contemplation, preparation, action, maintenance, and termination. This analysis of the change process takes into account movement forward and backward on this continuum. The model also outlines the types of psychotherapeutic approaches that are most effective at different stages.

The building blocks of change are ten processes, or types of activity, that occur within these six stages. These processes, found to a greater or lesser extent in all therapies, are: consciousness raising, self-liberation, social liberation, counterconditioning, stimulus control, self-reevaluation, environmental reevaluation, contingency management, dramatic relief, and helping relationships.

The FAM postulates that these ten change processes making up the activities of the various methods of psychotherapy can be reconsidered as four activities. Perhaps this may be best demonstrated by translating one stage of the TtM, with its typical therapeutic activities, into the FAM. Below is an attempt to do that with the first TtM model stage.

Client–therapist contact in the Precontemplation stage is not based on explicitly stated client self-change goals. Usually, contact with the therapist is related to an organizational demand, such as a requirement before returning to military duty or law-enforcement work. This contact is sometimes court mandated, especially because of drug or alcohol abuse. In Department of Veterans Affairs programs, it is *possible* to see clients in the Precontemplation stage because of the structure of the pension system. Veterans who have been psychologically disabled often must — or believe they must — "jump through the hoop," or go through the motions of psychotherapy in order to receive the pension they need for financial security, even if they believe the therapy to be ineffective in helping them.

According to the FAM model, clients in this stage most likely have associative networks containing the elements that others see as problems, or that they recognize as problems, but either do not intend to try to change, or believe are unchangeable. The reasons the client may not try are best illustrated by the beliefs or cognitive elements in the associative networks related to the "problem." Probably more common among nonveterans is: "There is nothing wrong with me, the world is crazy." Precontemplative combat veterans who retrospectively find themselves overreacting to threat or perceived threat, avoiding family, and having intrusive symptoms will more likely have beliefs such as: (1) "I'm powerless to change, even if I wanted to. The war has permanently branded me."; (2) "Change is dangerous because I would lose my edge and become vulnerable."; (3) "I deserve to suffer."; (4) "It's other people's fault I am like this. Let them change." (These and other beliefs are addressed later and in detail.) Some or all of these beliefs might be accessed as part of an associative network activated by stimuli associated with the "problem" area, or just change in general. Emotions that may be accessed as part of the same network could include sadness, anger, fear, resignation, numbness, and so on. Images may relate to trauma, or to others who have been seen in hopeless situations.

The therapeutic interventions the Transtheoreticians recommend at the Precontemplation stage (Prochaska and DiClemente, 1992; Prochaska, Norcross, and DiClemente 1994) highlight *consciousness-raising* statements to help the client become more aware of "causes, consequences, and cures of their problems" (Prochaska and DiClemente, p. 304). They point out that awareness is the primary change process of dynamic methods. The transtheoretical approach includes arenas or *levels of change* that one method or another might emphasize. At the Precontemplation stage, Adlerians are cited for work with maladaptive cognitions, Sullivanians for interpersonal conflicts, strategic therapists for family system conflicts, and analytic therapists for intrapersonal conflicts. It is also recognized that the symptom/situational level may be addressed, but no school is cited (Prochaska and DiClemente, p. 309) for its methods at this stage at that level.

The other TtM change process prominent at the Precontemplation stage is *social liberation*, referring to society's offer of help in solving the problem. Prochaska et al. (1994) use examples such as no-smoking rules in buildings helping people to consider quitting smoking. In FAM terms social liberation would be Category 1 and 2 activities.

FAM Understanding of Therapy

From the viewpoint of the four-activity model, the work of the Precontemplative stage depends on the specific content of the problem associative networks, and what needs to be added in order for the contained information to be thoroughly processed. If the client does not know that his dissatisfaction in life is related to his own behavior, such information must be introduced. If the client is aware of having a role in his discomfort, but believes he cannot change, then information to the contrary can be either introduced or accessed, such as through accessing memories of previous successful changes or known examples of people who have changed in similar situations. Every method of therapy — not just dynamic therapies — has its own explicit approach to informing the client that there is a path to change and the nature of that path.

It should be noted that nonverbal information is introduced or accessed in therapy, and perhaps it is the nonverbal aspects of the therapies Prochaska and DiClemente list at this stage that truly places them there. The nonjudgmental accepting attitude of the dynamic therapies, and of Roger's client-centered therapy, introduce or access information that the client is worth being with. When successfully transmitted, this attitude allows troubling information to be accessed and integrated with the new or reawakened information that the client is acceptable, leading to resolution of damaging aspects of the associative networks.

The FAM is in agreement with the TtM in that the ultimate goal of psychotherapy is to "...enable the individual to engage in more accurate information processing." What the FAM adds to the TtM is a more elemental understanding of the underlying process. The FAM conceptualizes therapy in terms of specific elements of the client's associative networks, and what explicitly the therapist can offer the client to change things there. If the client has the belief he is worthless, feels fear and habitually turns away from others, and has memories of the establishment of these responses, what does the therapist do to help the client access the networks that contain that information and integrate information into that network that will allow the damaging aspects of it, the emotion, the negative self-beliefs, and habits to process out, and to retain what is of value? How close do we sit? What facial expressions help? What words do we say, what do we ask the client to do? To understand and do therapy well from this point of view, it is necessary to borrow the activities of previously established methods. It may also be helpful to know which patterns of association are typical of a given situation, but at the same time ignore the confusion of theoretical structures built around these activities.

Lazarus' Multimodal Model of therapy, I think, is a more parsimonious conceptualization of the therapy process than the TtM and much more the precursor of the FAM. Lazarus' (1992, p. 236) stated goal, "...to reduce psychological suffering and promote personal growth as rapidly and as durably as possible," is not phrased in the information processing terms of the TtM, but his model is more directly translatable into information processing conceptualizations. He understands the client (human) situation in terms of its component parts: behavior, affect, sensation, imagery, cognition, interpersonal relationships, drugs/biology. He describes interventions aimed at specific elements in what I am referring to as associative networks. He is inclusive and integrative of the various therapy methods but rejects making his underlying belief in social and cognitive learning theory a part of his formal model.

The FAM includes a general level of abstraction of the therapy activity that Lazarus appears to intentionally avoid. In doing so, it is organized around the information processing activities the therapist tries to have the client engage in (for example, accessing, introducing) rather than the elements to be accessed, or introduced to be changed (for example, behavior, emotion) in the associative networks. While both levels of analysis make sense, the FAM allows for inclusion of Category 3 activity and better highlights the overlap among the various methods of psychotherapy.

In the end, for the most part, integrationists and nonintegrationists, we are observing the same phenomena. To again borrow a well-worn Buddhist metaphor: while it may look like we are all blindfolded and touching the elephant in different places, each proclaiming the primacy of our part, in fact we all have a pretty good idea of what *most* of the elephant is like. The real question has become: which language of considering the elephant is most useful for clinical practice and research? Of course, I think mine is, because I think it captures the full elephant and best integrates the parts the others have already noted.

chapter 4

Clinical Recommendations Prior to Category 3 Activity

In the previous chapter, the four-activity model was introduced and I attempted to explain how the activities of the various methods of therapy could be interpreted in the FAM. I hope it is clear that a specific intervention taken out of context will not distinguish a counselor who subscribes to the FAM from a counselor who doesn't. That is, asking a client to consider the similarities between his current and past work difficulties will involve the same conversation whether or not the therapist considers it a Category 1 activity. In the same way, people accurately predict that apples fall to Earth whether one subscribes to Newtonian physics, Einstein's theories, or the animistic view that apples embrace the Earth because they love it so. It's just that one model will take you farther in understanding and successfully intervening in a wider variety of situations.

Similarly, establishing a negative cognition in an EMDR session will be the same exercise whether or not the therapist considers this a Category 1 activity. In practice, use of the FAM may only be evident in the therapist's thinking when he or she notices that a client is not progressing in information processing. The therapist may then decide that an effective way through the block would be a new Category 3 activity, or perhaps a different Category 1 activity, such as asking the client to participate in an empty chair exercise instead of asking further questions to better access negative cognitions. Using the FAM in these situations may make the therapist's thinking more fluid and creative, while retaining coherence and ultimately being more helpful to the client.

I would now like to explore the specifics of EMDR and discuss its use in general, then in detail, in working with one of the most difficult psychological problems, the posttraumatic psychological responses of combat veterans. Because a specific intervention will be no different when done from the FAM model than when done from the model of the school that developed the type of intervention, as the discussion develops I will talk about the intervention and mention, but not dwell on, its relationship to the FAM model, which I hope will be self-evident anyway.

To return to the problems of combat veteran clients and begin with the use of the language of the AIP and four-activity models: the combat veteran has extensively elaborated associative information networks containing information that is experienced as visual images, behaviors, beliefs, emotions, odors, and so forth. Some of these elements are represented as powerfully as they can possibly be in humans, and occur many times. Beliefs may run the gamut from "I am going to die immediately," "I am purely evil," or "I am absolutely helpless," to "I am a God, I have the power of life and death," or "I am damned for eternity, with no hope of forgiveness." Sensations may include complete loss of self-control of bodily functions or excruciating pain. Behaviors may include lethal attacks or suicidal behavior.

According to the FAM model, therapeutic questions that may come up when processing is stalled are: How can the associative networks be accessed when clients have difficulty doing so? What new information might be introduced when processing is stalled? Which activities may best promote the processing of information, and what strategies should be considered to limit the accessing and processing of information when that is desired?

Exploring the treatment of combat-related trauma may be especially valuable, as it is generalizable to other sources of trauma in adolescents or adults. In combat, participants may take any, or all, of the three trauma roles: victim, observer, or initiator. Additionally, combatants are usually multiply traumatized with life-threatening situations, and often with physical injuries, so severity[1] is present. Combatants sometimes are in the dangerous situation voluntarily and sometimes involuntarily, so another important dimension is learned about.

In the previous review of the stages of EMDR, I briefly presented the stages as Shapiro does in her text and workshops. I will not try to repeat Shapiro's definitive explanations of these stages here; rather, I will offer some alternatives to the way information is considered in some of these stages. As one learns EMDR, I strongly suggest first mastering Shapiro's approach before considering the modifications shared herein.

Stages of Treatment

1. History and Treatment Planning

Every method of psychotherapy has this stage. In this, an advanced text, I am not going to instruct on history taking; Dr. Shapiro has covered this topic comprehensively in her text. I will suggest that an overview of the client's problems may be efficiently gained using Lazarus' Multimodal Inventory, with supplemental specific trauma history questions. It is

1. As Dollard and Miller (1950) point out, writing between World War II and the Korean War: "In combat and in infancy the extremes of hunger, fear helplessness, confusion and timeless strain are reproduced. Only in childhood and in combat are the individual's own capacity to control his life so meager and ineffectual." (p. 130) One may reasonably disagree about whether or not the list is limited to infancy and combat, but not, I think, with the content of the experiences.

irresponsible not to recommend extremely comprehensive history taking; however, most clinicians learn relatively quickly that history taking is never complete. This is especially true when helping clients with reactions to trauma, where the avoidance or denial of the events — or aspects of them — is a central feature of the problem. I have found that EMDR, in its powerful accessing of experiences often not otherwise available, profoundly clarifies the limits of initial history taking.

There is some belief that very few episodes are not recalled, and that clients suppress, rather than repress or dissociate, trauma (Karen, 1994). I tend to believe in both conscious and unconscious contributions to the missing history. I have had many clients who recall engaging in some bloody activity who are dumbfounded about why they would do such a thing. During the course of treatment, they then recall that their self-mortifying deed followed soon after some horrible loss of their own, a connection they had not realized since the event occurred. In these cases, it seemed unlikely that there would be a deliberate unwillingness to connect events that would lead to some mitigation of guilty feelings. In either case, combat clients will often not give history on their most important trauma. Consequently, over-adherence to too thorough a history can lead to the failure to promote the accelerated information processing that will lead to relief; better, less hostile functioning; and, by the way, a fuller history.

One addition to traditional history taking activity that I have found helpful for veterans and nonveterans is to get preliminary information about negative cognitions and the affect associated with potential target events as the client tells his or her story. For example, if a client comes for relief from distress following a rape, as she is describing the events, the therapist might ask her what thoughts she had about herself both as she experienced and as she described the events. The client's response usually should not be pursued and cognitions should not be refined at this point as they would be just prior to beginning Category 3 activity, but the area can be broached. Similarly, inquiry can be made as the client gives further history and relates other events, not necessarily traumatic, such as changing residence in childhood.

As to treatment planning: if EMDR incorporates a combination of the best accessing and teaching techniques of other methods, and adds an information processing facilitator, then treatment planning should almost universally include the recommendation to use EMDR relatively early in therapy. The question of whether to recommend it at a given time rests on whether there are some situations in which facilitation of information processing would be useless or even detrimental. Shapiro indicates that there are several circumstances in which this is the case. These can generally be described as situations in which accelerated facilitation may lead to overwhelming accessing that the client, even with good support, will find more damaging than productive. Examples include clients in fragile health for whom abreaction could be physically threatening, and clients with severe dissociative problems for whom Category 4 activity is needed to prevent dangerous decompensation.

Many clinicians expect some discussion of diagnostic categories in treatment planning with EMDR. And, in fact, Dr. Shapiro introduces and teaches the basis of EMDR in Level 1 and 2 training in terms of diagnostic categories. This was, and is, sensible for several reasons. One is that DSM-IV is the lingua franca of the mental health field and, if one is going to have something as radically new as EMDR seriously evaluated, it is best to use the accepted language and, generally, to violate as few traditions as possible.

In addition to acceptance, there is the learning strategy of taking on one piece at a time; it is to be expected that learning will take place most readily in the context of categories with which people are already familiar. Thus, in the beginning stages of learning, when a workshop participant asks, "What do you target when you use EMDR with PTSD?" it may be best to answer: "Have the client bring up a picture of the worst moment…" When a participant asks, "What do you target when you use EMDR with phobias?" it may be best to answer: "Have the client bring up a picture of the worst moment…." At an advanced level, the best answer might be to begin to deconstruct the diagnostic categories by replying, "Diagnosis doesn't give the most important information — identify, access, the events, and the information the client needs to process."[2] I am proposing, consistent with the traditions of behavioral analysis, that evaluation in terms of diagnostic category — as important as it may be economically or socially — is often superfluous for clinical evaluation and treatment planning. What needs to be identified are thoughts, images, feelings, and so on — stimuli and behaviors that are the problems — as well as thoughts and images that are preferred. Even though some practitioners of behavior therapy might not consider EMDR behavioral treatment, it calls for a return to the early behavioristic principle for specificity in problem definition, a position modern behaviorism has been shaped away from by a number of factors, notably the financial reinforcers used in the mental health industry and the value of borrowed "legitimacy" by using the medical model for psychological problems.

So, in evaluation and treatment planning, a primary discrimination is between problems that are learning based and may be amenable to resolution through the processing of information versus problems that involve a systematic biological dysfunction that will not respond to information processing approaches. I am careful how I use *biological*, because information processing is also a biological activity. It is probably safe to say that Attention Deficit Hyperactivity Disorder (ADHD) and Bipolar Affective Disorder are two problems involving biological factors that, at base, will not respond to information processing solutions. (It must be noted that symptoms of PTSD that are mistaken for these problems may be amenable to EMDR treatment.) Such clients may benefit remarkably from assistance in processing negative self-beliefs and emotions that come from difficulties they have had because

2. In Shapiro's second level training, there is emphasis on both the importance of recognizing the use of diagnostic categories and the value of thinking beyond these categories. In both the introductory and second level training, treatment protocols are offered by diagnostic category designed to make it likely that relevant information will be accessed.

of systemic biological problems; processing may thereby reduce the impact of the basic biological problems. So a person with ADHD who has the idea that she is worthless because she has difficulty learning in some situations may gain considerable relief if her belief can change to "Everybody's got problems, I'm wise not to judge myself or others." I am aware that readers may be surprised by the nature of this "improved" belief, expecting it to be something like "I'm a good person" or "I am worthwhile." My reasons for offering a seemingly less positive and certainly more complex belief have to do with the nature of self-judgment in general, which I will take up in greater detail when I discuss positive cognitions.

Medication

The effect of psychotropic medication on psychotherapy is not a new area of discussion; however, the effects of medication on accelerated information processing therapies is. All the available information is based on clinical observation. Some of these observations were collected in a survey I conducted of the first 1,600 clinicians to be trained in EMDR (Lipke, 1995); there were over 400 responses. One question in that survey asked: "From your experience, what effects do the use of medication or illicit drugs have on EMDR results?" (p. 383) Very few psychiatrists had taken EMDR training at that time; five who did reported EMDR to be unaffected by medication, but did not specify the medications used. One other reported that desipramine, a tricyclic antidepressant, did not seem to alter the effectiveness of EMDR. Of the psychologists surveyed, 12 reported that medication, in general, did not interfere with EMDR; 13 others were more specific, stating that antidepressants did not seem to cause problems. Three reported that antidepressants improved the effectiveness of EMDR. One reported that anxiolytics — minor tranquilizers — improved EMDR effectiveness. Twelve reported marked or some reduction of effect from medication in general. Six other respondents specified that nonantidepressants (four mentioned benzodiazapines) decreased the effectiveness of EMDR.

From these responses, as expected, the interaction between EMDR and medication appears complex. In reporting these results previously, I stated, "Overall these reports suggest medication does not rule out the use of EMDR and, in some cases, perhaps with severe depression, medication could provide sufficient stabilization to begin EMDR treatment." (p. 383) My personal clinical experience is consistent with this conclusion, except that I have had clients on major and minor tranquilizers with whom I have used EMDR to good effect. I suspect that these medications have somewhat limited the thoroughness of the EMDR response.

This point was illustrated by a client whom I will call Bob L.[3] Bob has long been treated with neuroleptic for psychotic symptoms, including the belief that others were monitoring his conversations. At the time I began his

3. For the sake of confidentiality, all clinical examples will be thoroughly laundered. Client names and details of events are changed so that incidents referred to are not identifiable.

psychotherapeutic treatment, he had been obsessively thinking about a recent episode when he was on a boat; he brandished a wrench, threatening to strike the boat of someone who had steered dangerously close. He also threatened the life of the man on that boat. Obsessively tormented over his behavior, he was adamant that he did not want to repeat it. We worked on the issue with EMDR to reprocesses this event and he was able to reduce his distress.

In the 3 years since then, Bob L. has engaged in no threats or acts of violence. This is not to suggest that EMDR resolved any concerns with violence, and it did not eliminate paranoid delusional thinking in general, but it does suggest that EMDR may be beneficial in treating these problems for a client on major tranquilizer medication.

This brings us to the question of how it is determined which problems have an underlying systemic biological base and which don't. ADHD, Bipolar Affective Disorder, and the problems we call schizophrenia likely have this base. However, other disorders ascribed a biological cause may not be as immutable. For example, I and other therapists have noted that the exaggerated startle response, a symptom of PTSD which has been ascribed to a possible permanent change, has diminished in some PTSD clients after successful treatment with EMDR.

In summary, for the nonpsychiatric psychotherapist, a diagnosis that indicates a biological problem whose symptoms are responsive to medication does not preclude at least some effectiveness from EMDR therapy. In addition, there are so many open questions about the etiology of problems that appear related to irreversible systemic causes that we may learn something about etiology, about what is and isn't truly biologically systemic, by watching client responses to EMDR.

Potential Negative Effects

As one client asked, "Doc, what's the downside? Everything has one." My response to this client was based on the practitioner survey mentioned above (Lipke, 1995). That survey indicated that 86% of the therapists found the emergence of repressed material to be more frequent with EMDR than other treatments they used. Similarly, 29% found EMDR led to in-session dissociation more often than other treatments, while 20% found in-session dissociation less often. However, 49% reported suicidal ideation and activity to be less frequent with EMDR; only 2% found it to be more frequent. And 32% reported postsession dissociation to be less frequent with EMDR, while only 14% found it to be more frequent. So we can suppose that within the therapeutic session, there may be an increase in discomfort for some clients, with a postsession decrease in discomfort.

My own clinical experience, working predominantly with Vietnam combat veterans, is similar to the report in the practitioner survey, except that I tend to get more reports of between-session difficulty. The reason for this, based on client reports and my clinical experience, is that combat veterans more frequently deal with multiple traumas, guilt, and fear of acting violently when emotionally aroused than most trauma victims — leading to more frequent interruption of the trauma work. I also must note that I have had a small minority of clients who began trauma work with EMDR, accessed extremely painful material, did not complete reprocessing in the session, refused further EMDR work, and subsequently had increased intrusive experiences, although exhibiting either no long-term regression of overall functioning or even improvement in other areas. For one of these clients, with both severe childhood and military trauma, the EMDR work was done on an inpatient basis. He volunteered for hospitalization because his trauma-based rage was nearly out of his control; he feared becoming violent, as he had in the past. We proceeded with EMDR in this controlled setting, the client dissociated, and hospitalization was continued for a few weeks. Further EMDR treatment was rejected. Some intrusive symptoms have persisted episodically at a severe level. However, he has shown some improvement in behavioral control and insight.

Client Education

Treatment planning means different things to different practitioners. Most would agree that it must be a collaborative process, requiring the therapist to inform the client of his or her way of thinking about the client's situation and available options, and the reasons for suggesting one alternative or another. Although I think this is important in all methods of therapy, many therapists can get away with deemphasizing explicit client education because their methods have face validity, or the education is the therapy. However, when one is recommending a treatment such as EMDR, which involves odd behavior, almost all clients will need — or should need — a sensible-sounding explanation. I recognize that there are clients who do not want the therapist to provide elaborate information; I ask these clients to indulge me anyway for at least the following reasons: (1) informed consent is not possible without information; (2) insisting on informing a client may access or introduce the notion that he or she is worthwhile and capable of understanding; (3) information reinforces the principle that our work is a partnership, in which the therapist is the junior partner, not an occult experience guided by a wizard.

This last point is best illustrated in EMDR when the client gets stuck while working toward complete processing of dysfunctional information and integration of appropriate positive information. By "stuck" I mean that information stops processing and the client remains uncomfortable and without change in content between sets of EM. When this occurs and simple changes in Category 3 activity do not advance processing, often the best intervention is to ask the client to explain what is causing the impasse. This is usually the most direct route to progress, much faster than the therapist "mystically" pulling interpretations and observations out of the air to access aspects of the client's associative networks that would produce progress. The more the client knows about the therapeutic process, the more likely he or she is to progress through difficult moments. And, again, asking this way accesses the notion that the client's opinion is important.

One way to emphasize the importance of sharing information is to supplement in-session explanation with written material. I have used the following handout with many clients.

Some Thoughts About Psychotherapy

— Howard Lipke, Ph.D.

This is meant to be a brief discussion of some very complicated ideas. Please use it to get a general idea of how psychotherapy works, and as the basis for questions and discussion.

When people consider beginning psychotherapy, it is usually because they have some very uncomfortable feelings, thoughts, and/or behavior. They may understand how these are connected to some part of their lives, or they may seem as though they come from nowhere. In either case, people come to therapy because they have some desire to have these change. For example, sometimes the change they desire is to have less painful feelings, or sometimes people say they "just want to understand" why they think, feel, or act the way they do.

Even though feelings, thoughts, and/or behavior are closely connected and profoundly affect each other, the work of improving them, in outpatient treatment, usually starts with either feelings or thoughts. (In inpatient treatment, because of the supervised setting, change can more frequently start with behavior.) Psychotherapies usually (but not always) focus on thoughts, which then may affect and improve feelings. Psychotherapists sometimes directly work with feelings, for example when they use relaxation exercises as part of therapy. Medication is sometimes used to try to affect feelings or behavior directly, which then influences thoughts in a positive way.

Where problem thoughts, feelings, and behaviors come from

From the point of view of the scientific psychologist, everything people think, feel, or do happens for reasons. Patterns of thoughts, feelings, or behavior are partly determined by hereditary factors and partly by life experience. Several overall tendencies may be strongly influenced by heredity; for example, a person's overall tendency to be excitable or reserved may be determined before birth. However, a person's excitability in a particular situation, or when in the vicinity of a particular person, will be almost completely influenced by experience. So, for example, no matter what a person's heredity, even many years after a military battle in which he was ambushed, almost anyone may have a strong, and maybe destructive, emotional reaction (feelings) to seeing a scene that reminds him of the battle. In addition, anyone may develop long-term changes in self-concept (thoughts) and behavior patterns based on that ambush.

Problem patterns of thinking, feeling, and behaving often get established in one of two ways (remember, there are also other ways to look at this; it is not an all-inclusive list):

1. *Through a very powerful or traumatic event*: for example, a child or adult who is beaten by a person in authority may develop a pattern of strong emotional response to authority. Depending upon the exact circumstances, the most obvious pattern of emotion displayed may be either anxiety or anger. A pattern of thinking may also develop in which everyone in authority is seen as evil or selfish. Or a pattern of thinking about the self may develop in which a person never tries to meet his or her goal because of the belief that he or she is weak and will be stopped by someone in authority. (Of course, multiple traumatic events have increased potential to cause problems.)

2. *Through less powerful but repetitive events, especially in childhood*: for example, it is not difficult to see how mild, lovingly intended, but constant criticism from an authority could lead to *some* of the same effects seen in the person who was beaten. For the person who is either criticized repeatedly or beaten, the problem feelings, thoughts, and behaviors may start as automatic reactions to the event. However, what starts as an automatic reaction may come to serve a purpose. The reactive acceptance of an authority's seeming judgment of incompetence, and the behavior reaction of avoidance of the authority, may turn into a long-term protective behavior pattern of never trying diligently to meet a goal. A person who learns to reactively accept the idea that she or he is incompetent, and never tries hard to meet a goal, may believe she or he won't

become *as* disappointed in failure because little effort was expended. So, thinking about herself or himself as incompetent and, therefore, not trying hard may become protective. This example uses mistreatment by authority to make a point. It should be noted that extended neglect or even too much attention could lead to problem patterns or, as they are sometimes called, schema.

Psychotherapy

Psychotherapy that starts with thoughts tries to identify the events the client has experienced, recognize patterns of thinking that the client has learned, examine pattern usefulness, and use the intellect to develop new understanding. These thinking changes may then lead to more comfortable feelings and more adaptive behavior. Sometimes, just identifying troublesome events is enough to begin positive change. Other times, when the patterns are very deeply experienced, it is necessary to work extensively with the events that produced the patterns. In either case, just identifying the patterns is not enough to make for lasting change; new ways of thinking have to be practiced if change is going to be permanent.

As mentioned above, sometimes psychotherapy starts to break patterns by focusing on changing feelings. Biofeedback, meditation, and relaxation training are some forms of this.

There is also a powerful kind of psychotherapy first written about in 1989 that, for many people, helps make changes in thinking and feeling at the same time. This is called Eye Movement Desensitization and Reprocessing (EMDR); it begins by having the client notice thoughts and feelings at the same time, and then engage in a physical activity, usually rapid eye movements, as guided by the therapist. Sometimes EMDR leads very quickly to emotional relief and better understanding of events. Sometimes EMDR first leads to intense emotion, or to thoughts of unexpected events that then lead to intense emotion. When this happens the client sometimes gets fearful that the therapy is not working or is making him worse. If the client can allow himself to continue, there will usually be a good therapeutic result. However, as with medication or other medical treatments, there is some risk. In the case of

EMDR, giving up in the middle of treatment increases the risk, just like climbing off the table in the middle of surgery would increase that risk.

No one is yet sure why EMDR is so powerful. The theory I think most likely true is that, when events that have strong negative emotion are stored in the brain, they are stored differently than other events. They are frozen and not integrated into the rest of experience. For example, a person who is nearly killed in a fire may always remember the fire in the same way with the same emotion that was there when the fire occurred. When she remembers the fire, she may think "I'm going to die" or "This is too horrible for me to bear." Somewhere in her brain she also knows that she is glad she survived and that she learned a lesson about life, but these more adaptive thoughts aren't connected to the memory of the fire because the images of the fire, including the thoughts about it, are frozen away from other information in the brain. Many scientists think that it is during the dreaming stage of sleep (rapid eye movement, or REM, sleep) that the brain "digests" memories of emotional events and connects the thoughts and feelings about those events to the rest of a person's knowledge (for example, connects the thought "I'm glad I survived"). For a variety of reasons, sometimes the dream stage of sleep doesn't accomplish this. It is thought that EMDR may serve the same function as the REM stage of sleep, and does it more efficiently because the person is awake and has the help of the therapist.

Even when EMDR works quickly and well, and helps to eliminate the painful effects of experiences from the past, clients still may need to develop new ways of dealing with the difficult situations that are part of even the most fortunate person's life. This part of psychotherapy often focuses on practicing new behaviors first, then working with the thoughts and feelings that are associated with new situations.

I hope this outline has been helpful to you in understanding the therapy process. It was not meant to be complete. Please use it as a jumping-off point to ask any questions you have about your situation or the therapy process.

This handout is neither all-inclusive nor a substitute for thorough discussion, but it does, I think, establish a base of knowledge and open up the process necessary for most effective counseling. Note that this handout may leave a client for whom EMDR is *not* immediately recommended wondering why it is not being offered. Obviously, I think therapy is better served by the clinician responding to this question directly, rather than avoiding it. With a client who I believe would likely stop in the middle of trauma work, or one who is not ready to entertain the negative self-thoughts that may come up, I will explain my concerns. I may tell a client that I am concerned that fully opening up their thoughts and feelings in some areas, before they develop a way of coping with the effects, may lead them to withdraw from the work and leave them feeling worse than when they started. If a client accuses the therapist of a lack of faith in his or her strength, I would certainly express my sympathy for their feelings and frustration that I cannot move faster, then explain that to do so would mean not having sufficient respect for their pain and, therefore, not behaving responsibly and competently. I find that it is rare for a client not to be responsive to honest acknowledgment of the client's pain and the therapist's limitations.

The version of this situation I find potentially most difficult is one in which the client reports being troubled by events I have good reason to believe did not occur, or occurred in a way substantially different than reported. In working with combat veterans, one must be very careful in confronting a client whose version of events differs from what appears probable, because sometimes the highly improbable has, in fact, occurred. Other factors that make confrontation potentially damaging are the fact that trauma victims, especially from combat, have already been hurt by societal neglect and outright rejection, as well as their own self-doubts. I have undoubtedly done EMDR with target material that was fabricated, and I did not know it; at times, neither did the client.

Neissen and Harsch (1992) have written interestingly on this point, demonstrating that emotion-related memory may be recalled accurately or inaccurately, almost irrespective of the subjective certainty of accuracy.

Finally, I have not mentioned what I think is the most important part of the treatment planning stage, the agreement to a contract. Extensive discussion of therapeutic contracts is not appropriate here, but I must mention that I believe that a preliminary contract, including the identification of problems to be addressed and the desired outcome, is a cornerstone of ethical and effective treatment. The initial appointment may end with only a contract to meet again and further discuss goals. Goals may be established before the educational steps take place, but should be considered for modification or reaffirmation after the educative discussion. The importance of goals becomes glaringly clear to me when I do a consultation: when a client is not making progress, I usually find (and the therapist readily agrees) that the therapist is not clear on client goals, or has goals different from those of the client.

2. Preparation

Some elements Shapiro covers in the preparation stage, such as the basic explanation of EMDR, was here covered in the history and treatment planning section. In addition to the suggestions made above, I may include technical material discussed in the scientific explanation of EMDR.

Coping with Increased Distress

At this stage of treatment, an essential feature is client preparedness to cope with increased distress that may occur between sessions. Many clients have relaxation, self-hypnosis, or meditation activities that they have used to manage acute stress. It is helpful to explore these and assess their value to the client. If the client does not have an effective method of stress management, it is important to teach one.

It should be noted that relaxation techniques can sometimes have the opposite effect and cause distress (Heide and Borkovec 1984). I have found that teaching relaxation per se at this stage is sometimes counterproductive with combat veterans and others who believe a high state of vigilance is essential for survival. Suggesting "relaxation" may be taken by the client as a sign the therapist does not understand the client's situation. So, at this stage of EMDR treatment I usually refer to "stress management methods" that may help the client control unneeded tension. I often include a discussion of arousal theory, the Yerkes/Dodson law, then briefly mention that scientific studies show that there are levels of arousal best for tasks of different levels of complexity and explain how excessive arousal or vigilance can lead to greater danger. I may compare optimal war zone/guard duty arousal, where the task is dangerous but simple and a high state of arousal is necessary, to peacetime arousal where a similarly high level is likely to lead to over-interpreting threat and creating a more dangerous situation. In this context I teach breathing exercises, such as alternate nostril breathing,[4] and other methods to help clients reach what they define as an optimal level of arousal.

Some EMDR therapists have reported success using "safe place" imagery, paired with a Category 3 activity, prior to beginning the next phase of treatment. When I use safe place imagery at this stage I do not pair it with Category 3 activity. Shapiro gives explicit directions for safe place creation in her text. I have found this helpful for some clients; however, many combat veterans cannot identify a safe place and find the procedure unhelpful or counterproductive.

Resistance to Beginning

This is a difficult area for me to address because I am uncomfortable talking clients into anything. When clients are frankly negative about EMDR, but I believe it may be very beneficial, I will generally, at the beginning and during the course of therapeutic conversation, address their specific objections. Included is information about EMDR and the alternative approaches, with a discussion of possible paths and outcomes of the various options.

4. An Eastern meditation method in which the subject blocks the left nostril and inhales deeply with the right; the subject then frees the left, blocks the right, and exhales with the left. The subject then inhales with the left and exhales with the right. The exercise continues, with the subject switching the blocked nostril after each exhale.

I may joke with a client that he will have to talk me into doing EMDR and, in fact, he may have to. A therapeutic situation I most dearly want to avoid is one in which a client who feels pressured into EMDR painfully abreacts, then refuses to continue EM to process through the distress.

Hypnosis

Some clients ask whether EMDR is hypnosis, and even object to it because they assume it is. After mentioning that it really isn't clear what hypnosis is from a scientific point of view, I usually respond by explaining that I see EMDR as being "unhypnosis." (I make it clear that this is my best guess, based on research and clinical experience.) I briefly discuss different memory systems in the brain and explain how events associated with strong negative emotions get stuck in one memory system and do not integrate with the rest of the brain's knowledge. So the target event(s) kind of hypnotizes the person: when he is focusing on it, the rest of his knowledge is blocked out, such as when a hypnotized person might be convinced he is on the stage at Carnegie Hall singing an opera, he has to block out all knowledge that this is not true. EMDR is "unhypnosis" in that it continually works toward connecting the "hypnotized" event to the rest of memory. To return to a trauma work example, if a person remembers a fire she was trapped in, instead of just feeling as if she is still trapped, the knowledge that it is over and that she is safe can be connected to the memory of the event; thus, she can be relieved that it is over, instead of terrorized by the feeling that she is still in it.

I might also draw the further distinction that in hypnosis the client, while hypnotized, does the trauma work in that state; then, when dehypnotized, the client and therapist hope that the information experienced in the hypnotized state will integrate.

To relate this back to the four-activity model and declarative and non-declarative memory systems: when target material in nondeclarative memory storage is accessed hypnotically, substantial aspects of the experience are suppressed. The hypnotherapist works with the material in this state; then, after terminating the trance, the therapist, in effect, hopes that there will be integration between memory systems because of changes effected while the client was in the hypnotic state. In contrast, in EMDR the therapist helps the client access material in nondeclarative memory, then — instead of working with the material in that state — uses Category 3 activity to continuously facilitate the integration of information networks across memory systems. In hypnosis terms, the client when accessing the target material is brought close to *trance/dissociation*, but is continually kept from entering trance/dissociation by the Category 3 activity. I conceptualize therapeutic hypnotherapy as a combination of Category 1 and Category 4 activity.

Similarly, when addictions or unwanted behavior are treated with hypnosis, the therapist tries to teach the client to partially dissociate when she feels the urge to engage in the target behavior. Thus, when the client — in the course of normal activity — accesses the urge to engage in the undesired behavior, the urge becomes dissociated, perhaps through learned connection to nondeclarative memory. Given enough time and repetitions of this process, she may integrate the knowledge that, for example, cigarettes are not to be expected when you talk on the phone; then the urge is no longer dissociated, it is just no longer present. I will discuss this further when I address the use of EMDR with substance abuse.

Trying out EM or other activity is part of the preparation stage. Different types of Category 3 activity were described in some detail in Chapter 3. A client may have difficulty with EM, despite claims that he is trying. Sometimes such clients can be helped by doing a single EM, then two EM, and so on. Remember the long, fast sweeps are not necessary; some clients who cannot do this still benefit. Occasionally, a client cannot tolerate a hand sweeping across his face: in this case, place your hands on either side of his field of vision and alternately raise a finger on each hand or, as a majority of my clients prefer, use blinking electric lights. As mentioned, other procedures that have also been successful have not involved eye movement. In some cases it may be advisable to alternately tap the client's palms or the sides of his hands as they rest on his knees, or to snap your fingers alternately in the right and left ear. I have found alternate hand tapping to be somewhat gentler and preferable for clients who have unwanted strong, protracted, emotional responses. It may turn out that hand tapping, or the client tapping his own knees, will be the intervention of choice for fragile clients who cannot tolerate being touched by the therapist.

Examples from the Client's Past

Sometimes client resistance comes from the belief that it is a futile effort to try to "reprocess" an event from the past, so he doesn't want to suffer the discomfort of targeting the painful event. Such a client may be asked if he can remember an incident from childhood in which a friendship didn't work out, or a game was lost, and how devastating that was at the time but now it brings up no distress, or may even seem funny or purely educational. The client is asked to consider what happened to the emotion from that event.

In this situation, I might teach the client the SUD scale and use this phrasing: "Think back to a time in high school or basic training when something bothered you quite a bit then, but doesn't bother you too much now when you think of it. On that 0 to 10 scale, with 10 most distressing, what number would you have given yourself at the time that event happened? What rating do you give yourself now when you think about it? What SUD rating would you give yourself when the (insert target to be worked on in therapy) was happening? What SUD rating do you give yourself now when you think of it?" The therapist might then add something like: "It is natural for the brain to digest that emotion so that the event is remembered as a memory, not reexperienced as if it is still happening. The purpose of this therapy is to help your brain experience that event as a memory." This may be a good time to mention the REM sleep hypothesis: that the brain may accomplish this in REM sleep, and that sleep disturbance may be due to wakening from the dream where this was supposed to be accomplished, because of the amount of distress. Thus the wakening stops the natural processing, which can proceed during EMDR because the person can choose to keep at it while awake and assisted by the therapist.

Resistance centered around the client's belief in the appropriateness of relief on the target issue may be met at this point. If this kind of resistance comes up, it is good to have it out in the open early. Ways of handling this resistance will be dealt with later.

Metaphors

The discussion about memory systems has been conducted in language designed for therapists and scientists; it may or may not be helpful to clients. I suppose that when it is helpful, it is accessing information networks that include the cognitive information, "I know what is going on, and it is good," as well as emotion and other information that goes along with that. For most clients, it is more helpful if they also access metaphors.

Shapiro offers simple and direct metaphors, including that the client is on a train moving down the tracks, "just noticing" the remembered events. Or that going through past events is like moving through a tunnel, reinforcing the idea of continually moving forward, which allows the encouraging words, "just move through it," spoken while the client is moving his eyes, to make sense.

More complex metaphors are sometimes helpful in client preparation. A useful one is the memory of being in an airplane circling, trying to land: landing represents bringing to consciousness, and going into the hangar represents desensitization. Before treatment, the most available memory at a given time begins to land (reach consciousness), but it is so painful that it is sent back up into the air (repressed). With EMDR treatment, the memory is aided in landing, which still may be painful, then it is parked in the hangar (desensitized). Even when this process is completely successful, the pain may not be gone because there are other airplanes to land and these may contain even more painful memories.

I assure my clients that the same technique that landed and parked the first memories can be successful with subsequent memories, but I let them know they must be aware of the prospects of discomfort. I also make sure they know that it may take more than one session to deal with each memory and, between sessions, they might still have strong negative responses, or more negative responses than they were having in the days prior to this work. At this point, I may remind them that they are in treatment because they are already having dissociative experiences and/or distressing thoughts and feelings, which are uninvited and destructive: if they do have a dissociative experience, at least it will be part of a process that is helping them no longer have such experiences.

3. Assessment

> "If you bring forth what is within you, what you bring forth
> will save you. If you do not bring forth what is within you,
> what you do not bring forth will destroy you."
> — Jesus, the *Gospel of St. Thomas* (Pagels 1979, p. 126)

Accessing the associative networks is the core of the assessment stage of treatment. Even though I often ask questions about cognitions and emotions that are part of this stage earlier, as part of my history taking and problem identification, by the time Category 3 activity is ready to begin, components may have already changed, so the elements are again identified. In simple situations, accessing the visual image, negative cognition, emotions, and feeling are the key to successful work. Although not the preferred method, it is even true that accessing one aspect of the dysfunctional network is often enough to begin ultimately successful processing of the whole network, as the naturally flowing chain of associations and Category 3 activity keeps accessing going. Clinically, this is seen when the beginning phases of accessing lead to strong emotion, which should be taken as a signal to begin Category 3 activity, rather than continue with therapist-led accessing.[5] With other clients, the accessing must be thorough to overcome the inhibition that arises to avoid the pain that accessing entails. Since clients often find superior positive cognitions as processing proceeds, it may also be thought that establishing the positive cognition before processing begins is not essential. However, it is difficult to determine in advance which situations do not require access of all elements, so full accessing is strongly recommended.

I think it is most beneficial to conceptualize accessing in broad terms, in two categories: (1) the dysfunctional network, with high nondeclarative memory involvement, and (2) the information that may be brought to the task of processing the dysfunctional network. The positive information is usually declarative and usually accessed through the positive cognition. I will refer to the potentially curative information as being part of a positive associative network, of which one element may be a positive cognition. Just as the dysfunctional network contains cognitions, visual images, emotions, thoughts, sensations (often combined in subnetworks sometimes labeled *schema*), the positive associative network may contain not only thoughts but visual images, emotions, and so forth, which may be combined into what we will call here *positive schema* (sometimes labeled ego ideals or archetypes).

The introduction of the positive cognition with its limits, before Category 3 activity begins, is usually preferable to accessing a full positive associative network, because full accessing may just become a Category 4 activity and prevent necessary accessing of the negative associative network. However,

---

5. Category 3 activity begins in response to accessing strong emotion *only* if it occurs in this stage of treatment, after history taking, education, and so on.

work with full positive associative networks may be valuable initially if the client does not have sufficient strengths to even begin accelerated processing of negative material. Positive schema will be discussed more fully later.

Up to this point in the discussion of assessment we have been focusing on accessing curative information that is already stored somewhere by the client. However, for many clients the information needed to be added to the negative associative network may not be present or, if present, may be weakly represented. This is where Category 2 activity, the introduction of new information, is particularly important.

In the following discussion of assessment process, I will refer to two basic strategies to be used in focusing the client's accessing: (1) working on the dysfunctional network, and (2) working on the positive associative network.

The Dysfunctional Network

In EMDR, the dysfunctional network is usually accessed in this order: visual image, cognition, emotion, and distressing body sensation. The visual image goes first because it is the most specific to a target situation, as well as concrete, so it is an easy marker of the target. Occasionally, clients have no visual image to target. Common reasons are dissociation of the visual aspect of the experience and simple lack of presence of visual stimuli during a target event. In a situation where there could be a problem with "false memories," I will ask the client to proceed without the visual aspect of the target. When this is not an issue, I may ask the client to construct a visual representation; that is, to make an internal artistic creation to represent the target situation.

Accessing the dysfunctional network through the emotions or body sensations is relatively straightforward compared to accessing cognitions. One problem that often arises with accessing emotion, especially in trauma cases, is that clients, especially combat veterans, will not recognize the presence of any emotion except anger. One form this failure to recognize takes is that, when the client is asked to identify the emotion, he states a belief and calls it a feeling. Clients may say something like: "I felt I was disrespected," or "I felt I was almost killed." The first thing the therapist can do in response to this is simply give brief instruction about emotion. Usually clients will understand. An efficient way to clarify and still validate the client's experience is to ask "And, when someone shows you disrespect, what is the name of the emotion or emotions that come to you? Sadness? Anger? Fear? Frustration?"

Clients who report being completely numb or emotionless when considering the target may find the accelerated part of the work of EMDR to be too threatening; extensive rapport work and clarification of the possibility of powerful emotion occurring should be considered before proceeding. Clients who have difficulty understanding the concepts will probably benefit from some education work. A group therapy format, easily modifiable for individual use to deal with the problem of emotion identification, is offered as a bonus in Appendix 1. Even when it is not used in an EMDR context, my clinical impression and the reports of many clients confirm that identifying and stating emotions is helpful.

I recognize that extensive warnings about the possibility of unpleasant experience may decrease the probability of effective processing; however, especially in working with combat veterans, the appearance of unexpected overwhelming images and emotion can lead to dangerous defensive reactions and, at the least, harm the therapeutic process. This is not a risk worth taking.

Cognitions

I would like to return to accessing the cognitive beliefs aspect of the target network and address it in greater depth. This emphasis is due to the relative complexity of this aspect, and the historical importance of cognition in psychotherapy; also, participants in EMDR training have the most trouble with this aspect of accessing.

The Negative

The first source of difficulty in establishing the negative cognition, paralleling the previously addressed problem with emotion identification, is that very often thoughts are referred to as emotions. Sometimes processing may proceed despite poor identification of cognition because the target network is fully enough accessed, but often this kind of language mixup causes or exacerbates an accessing problem. For example, when a client reports "I was angry," it is a good idea to elicit a cognitive statement by asking something like "As you feel this anger now, what *belief* about yourself or the world comes to mind?" I also explain to the client why it is important to distinguish between cognition and emotion. I find it helpful to therapy when clients learn that when the distinction is made, thoughts can then more easily be seen as hypotheses, which allows a greater chance for modification.

This distinction is an important part of my client consultation. It can be explained that thoughts and feelings go together and, although they always influence each other, for change to take place they have to be looked at separately. The example of a car speeding toward a collision with a post may be helpful. The collision will occur because of *both* the car's speed and direction together; however, preventing the collision will call for *separate* actions to adjust the speed and the direction. Similarly, if a person is going to adjust his course he will do best if he can identify and work on the thought and feeling functions separately for a time before, as he must, bringing them together.

Another basic source of difficulty is when the client chooses a negative cognition that was present at the time of the target event, or one that describes the action. Either of these may accurately fit the description of the thoughts occurring as the target is accessed in the present. However, neither is as likely to effectively help fully access the target network and to produce as generalized an effect, as the more global negative cognitions. For the few clients who have relatively simple, straightforward complaints and goals, who deny the relevance of a more global cognition, and are not easily persuaded to search for one, it may be more beneficial to start with what they do initially produce. If processing subsequently reaches an impasse, the therapist may be in a better position to work cooperatively with them on the issues of negative cognitions.

Half of several comprehensive methods of therapy — Rational-emotive Behavior Therapy (REBT), Cognitive Behavior Therapy (CBT), and Schema Focused Therapy (SFT) — may be viewed as studying the art of accessing the negative cognition. Ellis (1995) refers to negative cognitions as irrational beliefs that lead to the consequence of pervasive negative emotion. Young's (1990) Schema Focused Therapy helps the client to access patterns of beliefs that pervade and limit functioning. The development of the negative cognition in EMDR can benefit from consideration of techniques used by these and other therapists. However, tempting as it may be to maintain therapeutic conversation,[6] it is important not to turn an EMDR session into CBT or REBT therapy.

As Shapiro first developed the cognitive aspect of EMDR, she referred to the negative cognition as the "present cognition"; that is, the thought or belief that popped into the client's mind when a target situation was accessed. Given the client's negative definition of the situation, the cognition would, of course, be negative. Take, for example, a client remembering a robbery in which she was almost killed. Many true thoughts could come to a person in the exact same situation with the exact same outcome. If this client, when recalling the worst moment, thinks:

1. "I'm glad that is over," the likely accompanying emotion will be relief.[7]
2. "I survived that. Maybe I'm pretty tough," is associated with pride.
3. "That robber shouldn't have attacked me. I have the right to go to the store," is associated with anger.
4. "I'm going to die now," is usually associated with fear.

People who think (1) or (2) probably will not come for therapy. People who think (3) might. And we certainly hope those people who dwell on (4) show up for counseling. Because it is current beliefs that are associated with emotional response, the "present" is almost interchangeable with "negative" in considering the cognitive aspect of the network.

In order to recognize the ongoing influence of the event and maximize the therapeutic power of the cognition in accessing the network, Shapiro asks

6. Some therapists have reported that they don't use much EMDR because they like talking to their clients. I have observed therapists, in EMDR training sessions, avoiding starting Category 3 activity because they seemed to want to continue discussion, clarifying just one more point.
7. I won't argue whether the emotion or cognition comes first; either way, they do influence each other.

that when the negative cognition is formulated by the client in the past tense, it be put in the present tense. To reconsider the (4) cognition above, fearful clients sometimes offer maladaptive past-tense responses, such as "I almost died," which they dwell on over and over. If the cognition is "I almost died," we can see there is no reason to believe the memory would not access relief because the person wasn't killed. It is only through the maintenance of the belief as an active threat, in the present tense, that there is reason for active fear. So we may ask the client to consider putting this statement in the present tense. A cognition such as "I must be intensely on guard all the time, because I almost died," may evolve out of this effort to more powerfully access the negative associative network and make processing more likely.

My work with combat veterans has often illustrated the role of cognition in the processing of dysfunctional networks. On the average, I find clients with combat trauma to develop more therapeutic resistance, and to benefit more slowly, than clients with other types of traumatic experiences. I think this is partly due to the total amount of trauma that occurs with combat duty, partly due to the nature of the trauma and the virulence of the negative self-beliefs that arise from combat events. In combat, one is party to activities that are accepted and rewarded by authority in that context, but which in other contexts result in vilification by that same authority. Some people who have been in combat, and acted according to the norm of their situation, when accessing the dysfunctional network, may not only call themselves overtly or covertly (unconsciously), murderers, baby killers, cowards, Nazis (I had more than one client overtly say this), but also partly believe they deserve to be punished in the gruesome ways they believe or believed others (whom they had called the same names in another context) deserved to be punished. These thoughts are all part of the combat associative network for many veterans. And, understandably, this cognitive material can be difficult to fully access, even when other aspects of the network are available.

The personality theorist George Kelly (1955) had a method useful in helping clients access cognitions that, if accessed indelicately, can lead to overwhelming emotion and the disruption of rapport (accessing too much). Kelly called his approach the Personal Construct Theory. For Kelly, people act as scientists in the world, developing constructs based on evidence. But no construct occurs in a vacuum; if one develops, for example, the construct, label, or idea (these words can be interchangeable) of "intelligent" and puts a selected individual or himself into the category "intelligent," we can't know what the label fully means until we know what the alternative category is (Kelly posited that categories were always dichotomous). The simple definition could be that the alternative or contrast category is "everything else," or "nonintelligence"; however, people are more refined than that. To some people, "intelligent" implies different from "average"; to others, being "intelligent" implies different from "stupid"; and to others it means different than "sensible."[8]

---

8. The label on the contrast pole may also vary by situation.

It may also be interesting to consider that it is through pathways theorized by Kelly that following chains of negative associations may lead to integrating positive material, even when the positive material is not independently accessed through the positive cognition phase of EMDR. By this thinking, accessing the negative automatically partially accesses its "opposite," which then, as Category 3 activity proceeds, may itself become dominant in the associative network.

I first found Kelly's conceptualization helpful in work with a successful businessman on his discomfort with a disturbing childhood memory in which he was left alone in the dark.[9] The client was quite proud of his collection of motorcycles, and his skill in racing them. His initial work with the childhood incident in an EMDR session included a negative cognition around vulnerability. He achieved considerable desensitization, reducing his SUD level to 2 or 3, but it was clear that he was still troubled by the event, and he made no further movement to a variety of standard interventions. When asked, he said he didn't know what was keeping his discomfort level from completely reducing when he contemplated these past events. Given that the target events were around fear, and that his hobby included coura-geous behavior, I asked him about fear in general, and whether or not he ever questioned his own courage. He said, based on his behavior, that he didn't. I try to be delicate in these matters, out of respect for the solution the client has been using to manage painful material prior to therapy, and in order to maintain rapport. So, I explained George Kelly's thinking about how people experience the world:

> One theory of how we make judgments is that there is the judgment we make, such as calling ourselves or someone else intelligent or strong, but then there is a sometimes hidden comparison that we don't state. So when we call ourselves intelligent, we may mean "compared to average," or we may mean "compared to stupid." That unspoken comparison is very impor-tant, because if something happens that makes us think we are not intelligent, what we might mean down deep is stupid. When we rate ourselves we may fully believe that we fall in the positive category, but are still be concerned that somehow we could fall into the alter-native. You said that the belief that goes with your childhood incident is vulnerability. I wonder if there might be another belief, not that you have it, but that it comes up as a logical necessity because of the way that you think about courage. If, for you, the contrast

9. Because it occurred in the middle of the session, after Category 3 activity began, this inter-vention would normally be considered a cognitive interweave, not the establishment of a negative cognition; however, the form of establishing it was so like that of establishing a negative cognition that I applied it here.

> to courage is cowardice, you might think about that as
> you visualize the target incident.

Then I asked the client to do eye movements. The result was an immediate decrease in tension and the full recognition that he had behaved acceptably as a child.

It was not so important that this client use the specific negative cognition, "I am a coward"; the essential feature seemed to be that he allowed himself to access the construct. There are areas some clients will not enter without guidance, and often we will have to deduce what these are and help the client get there. To make this general point, I have sometimes told clients that the strategy of pushing painful thoughts away (Category 4 activity) may lead to temporary relief and it may be a good strategy while you are in the middle of dealing with the day-to-day events of life, but things that are pushed away keep coming back. It is only after the thing is let in and examined thoroughly that it may be put in its proper place.

If you access the network you can process it. If you don't, the fight you put up against accessing it will — if not destroy you — at least keep you from being able to fulfill your potential.

The Positive

After attempting to partially access the target, or negative associative network, through a visual image and negative cognition, Shapiro pauses to have clients identify the preferred or positive cognition. The cognition is rated for emotional believability and then, in most situations, not invoked by the therapist until the end of the work on the target network. As eye movement or other Category 3 activity proceeds, it is common for clients to spontaneously produce better positive cognitions, along with pictorial images, emotions, and sensations which appear to merge with and transform the target network.

The positive cognition accessed a few moments before Category 3 activity is to begin is one of several ways in which the positive associations are accessed to (it is hoped) integrate with the dysfunctional target material. During the course of information processing when clients are "stuck," often with strong emotional distress, positive material is invoked by the therapist in what Shapiro has called the "cognitive interweave." Since, as discussed previously with the positive cognition/schema, the "cognitive interweave" often contains nonsemantic elements, such as soothing images of a beloved support figure, I will refer to this aspect of treatment as the "interweave" without the word cognitive.

Shapiro clearly recognizes the importance of not only following the client in positive associations, but also of the therapist invoking noncognitive positive phenomena; however, she has not formally incorporated these concepts in the assessment phase. As Shapiro has developed EMDR, the positive network is not yet fully fleshed out at the assessment stage. Pieces of it are applied and/or developed as needed for each individual client. As mentioned earlier, I think it may be more beneficial to think of the positive cognition from the start as just one element of a positive associative network, more heavily weighted toward declarative than nondeclarative elements, that combine with the negative network in the resolution of trauma.

I have found that the more complex the client's situation is, the more important accessing or creating positive elements becomes. Because of the helpfulness of images in promoting it, I think it may be useful to add to this aspect of EMDR procedure, moving from positive or preferred cognition to the more general notion of *positive associative network* (PAN), containing subnetworks that can be referred to as positive schema. A positive schema, when identified before the initiation of Category 3 activity, could be limited to the traditionally sought positive cognitions, such as "I'm a capable person" or "It's in the past," or the positive schema could consist of images of ego ideals or spiritual beliefs — options that will be elaborated on in a later section.

"Problem" and "Solution"

As if there were not already enough added in here, another way to conceptualize the positive cognition or schema is to consider it the potential "solution." In this conceptualization, the "problem" is the negative associative network. This network stores information that, when active, causes *excessive* pain and dysfunctional behavior. In a sense, then, the negative network contains a problem that needs a solution. The solution is the positive material that may be added to this network, allowing its dysfunctional aspects, chiefly the overwhelming emotion or vivid visual images, to exit. As I describe the process of identifying the positive cognition or schema, I will sometimes refer to this as "finding the solution." Referring to the positive as the solution, as in "the solution to the problem of finding a way to make peace with an event," is sometimes valuable clinically, as well as conceptually. Thinking in terms of solutions may access less initial resistance than trying to have the client find something positive in a trauma. However, the idea of a solution may also present problems.

Rando (1993), in her extensive work on grief and mourning, discusses the problem of the client's acceptance of change in her extensive work on grief and mourning. She also makes the point that, while the person suffering loss may in fact be stronger or have somehow grown from it, it is inappropriate to consider loss itself as a problem that can be solved. She uses the term *accommodation*, similar to the way Piaget did in discussing human development, to describe the adaptive changes a person may make in responding to loss. I agree with her, but find that in clinical practice, while the client is acutely suffering with emotion and dysfunctionally negative thoughts, the word "solution" seems to fit, as long as it is clear that *solution* refers only to the dysfunctional aspect of the painful schema.

Before further elaboration on the idea of positive schema or solutions, it may first be worthwhile to more thoroughly address the roots of these ideas in EMDR, the positive cognition.

Positive vs. Preferred Cognition

The positive cognition was originally referred to as the preferred cognition, in the same way the negative cognition started as present cognition. For the sake of clarity it was almost always necessary to describe the preferred cognition as positive. Eventually, it is just easier to ask for the positive cognition in the first place. The move to the word positive is also consistent with Bandura's (1989) thinking and research about self-efficacy.

There are two concerns about the use of "positive" instead of "preferred," both of which Shapiro recognizes. First, rapport may be damaged if the client believes the therapist, in looking for a positive cognition, doesn't understand the depths of his loss or despair. In this situation, the word *preferred* conveys a more sympathetic message. Secondly, despite working on strong positive cognitions in the assessment stage, clients very often spontaneously produce more neutral-sounding, but obviously deeply satisfying, cognitions such as "It's over," stated with a sigh of relief. It is generally more acceptable in clinical practice to accept a positive cognition that does not meet the best standards than to push the client to see a solution that seems impossible, which undermines the credibility of the therapist as an empathetic listener. Therapists, therefore, must be prepared to accept the more limited solution, even though it may not seem like a positive cognition. So, while the term *positive* is used, the spirit of *preferred* should be maintained.

Regardless of how it is referred to, clients sometimes have problems when asked for an alternative to the negative cognition. Often clients fail to comply because they believe that their current thoughts or, more precisely, judgments are the only possibilities — which is, of course, part of the problem that brought them for therapy. In these situations I try to do a brief REBT-style intervention, which is probably Category 2 activity. I explain that there are many true thoughts about any given situation. Sometimes I start by giving an example of something innocuous, such as asking if the desert is sunny or if it is hot. When they say it is both, I explain that often one thought is dominant about a situation and that the thought that is focused on will often greatly affect how a situation affects us. With some clients, I may then give another example of a more closely relevant powerful situation, but one that is not their own so that I am not seen as overly influencing their selection of a preferred cognition. I might say:

> To pick something traumatic, let's say you had a friend
> die near you in a battle. It may be true that if you acted
> differently, he might be alive, so the words that come
> to you when you think about this might be "It was my
> fault." But it may also be true that you did the best
> you could under the circumstances, so the words that
> might come to you when you think about this would

be, "I was young and scared; he knows I did the best I could."[10] Both of these thoughts may be true. Which would you rather have come to you when you think about this situation? Which words would be helpful in having a positive life?

Then I ask the client to consider choosing his own positive cognition for his target event, to choose words he would prefer, words that could be true even if he doesn't fully accept them.

Sometimes clients object to the notion of finding a positive cognition because of the specific belief that any construction of an event that is not negative is a rationalization, and therefore "bullshit." When this occurs I sometimes engage the client in a discussion of causality, and the complexity of it. In the course of this discussion, I may ask the client the source of his knowledge that is blocking consideration of the positive cognition. Using this approach introduces or accesses the position that beliefs are learned and therefore subject to change:

THERAPIST: Where do you think you learned that explanations involving more complex understanding of responsibility were rationalizations or bullshit?

CLIENT: From my father, from the Marines.

THERAPIST: Did they have any self-interest in teaching you that causality was simple?

CLIENT: What do you mean?

THERAPIST: I mean, taking the Marines for example, wasn't their goal to teach you to not think too much and follow orders?

CLIENT: Were you a Marine?

THERAPIST: No, but I've met a lot of them. And from what I can gather, the military has to teach you to go risk your life. To get people to do that, they have to teach them not to think too much. One way to do that is to look at things very simply and call anything but self-blame for "mistakes" bullshit. You can see why this would also make life easier for a parent or anyone else trying to control behavior.

---

10. One must be extremely careful in using the "best I could" solution because the client may have some second thoughts about this that he is withholding. Also note that this is an example of a "less positive," past, rather than current, referent cognition that can be superseded later as some processing occurs.

CLIENT: Now that you mention it, it does make some sense. But sometimes it is just your fault.

THERAPIST: Yeah, we often do have some vital link in it when things go wrong — but this doesn't mean we shouldn't attempt to understand the complexity and use that knowledge to learn. So what thought could allow for a different, more valuable understanding of this event?

It may turn out that the information uncovered in this search will lead to a new target for processing. This target may involve situations in which skewed standards of gender role were acquired, and may become the first target processed, even before the "traumatic event" initially selected.

Sometimes clients choose as a positive cognition the thought that the event didn't happen at all. When this occurs I explain that, although we can't change history we can change how it affects our lives, and then briefly explain some basics of rational emotive behavior therapy. I also make it clear to the client the difference between memory and reliving. Clients are often ambivalent about memory of the trauma, or feel very strongly that it not be erased. I will discuses this further in a later section on desensitization and resistance.

There are a number of standard positive cognitions, often offered by clients spontaneously, and listed in EMDR manuals, that are potentially useful; however, when applied indiscriminately they may lead to problems in complete processing. Any cognition that implies — or that the client takes to mean — complete and permanent resolution of a problem, or achieving an impossible level of certainty or perfection, has a good chance of leading to incomplete processing. For example, when clients offer the positive cognition "I'm in control," there may be an underlying belief that the client is in complete control, and can never be out of control of a situation. Therefore, I ask if being in control implies perfection, that no matter what happens they can control things, or does it mean that they have a lot of options they can try to solve problems as they come up? I try (or, perhaps, can't help) making my response a little wordy so clients are provided some examples of possible changes and haven't been given a succinct positive cognition; they must make some choice in creating it. If the client persists in an impossible positive cognition, I will not expect that we will quickly get through the evaluation phase and get to Category 3 activity in that session. In this situation the therapeutic contract, in terms of goals, must be readdressed.

A good example of how a positive cognition got in the way of complete processing occurred with a client who was working on feelings related to a medical problem that was resolved, but still troubled her when she thought about the procedures used. She succeeded in reducing her SUD level to 2, but could move no farther. She showed no gain when she was asked to think of the positive cognition and do EM. Her positive cognition had been "I'm OK." I asked her if her positive cognition implied that her problem could never come back, or that she would have no more medical problems. She thought, then said perhaps it did mean she would have no more medical problems. She changed her positive cognition to: "I'm feeling OK right now, and I can enjoy that." We did a set of EM with that cognition and her anxiety resolved. In addition to being a good example to explain the clinical application of a specific principle, it also suggests the theoretical point that processing is the merging of associative networks, not simply desensitization.

Thinking of the positive cognition in its initial form, as the preferred cognition, also has another benefit; it allows for, and sometimes invites, reconsideration of self-rating in general. As suggested by research and theoretical writing on self-focused attention, ratings and evaluation of the self — when taken to excess — may be associated with psychopathology (Ingram, 1990; Wolfe, 1992). The defocus from the self is also suggested by an ancient tradition of Buddhist and Taoist philosophical thinking. Among modern writers, Watts (1961) and Linehan (1993) do wonderful work in exploring this theme in psychotherapy.

In working with discrete issues, where the client's goal is solely to be less troubled by a specific event, and this broader issue is bringing more to the treatment than the client is requesting, it falls outside the therapeutic contract. So if the client chooses a preferred cognition that is generally evaluative, appropriate, and positive, such as "I'm an OK person," as long as there is no implication of perfection, I may not raise the general issue of self-rating. If, on the other hand, there are multiple concerns, multiple trauma, and strongly developed and pervasive negative self-cognitions, the more general issues will inevitably be raised, and teaching about self-rating will be needed. In this regard, sometimes I convey to my clients that there are basically three ways to think about oneself, in ascending order of adaptiveness: negatively, positively, and nonjudgmentally. I discuss with them the fact that we humans cannot help but think about ourselves in each of these categories at times, but stress the importance of learning to emphasize the more adaptive end of the trio.

It seems that work with the positive cognition is the most underrated aspect of EMDR. It is probably the element most often skipped by therapists, for several reasons: one is that, after being established, the positive cognition is ignored in many treatment sessions, even when Shapiro's protocol is being followed rigorously, until the end, when the bulk of the work is done. (Bringing it up and then ignoring it is similar to an attorney who knowingly brings up an unacceptable point and then quickly retracts it, but the damage — or, in the case of therapy, the good — has been done.) Another reason is that clients often spontaneously improve positive cognitions during processing, so therapists may not want to "waste" the effort developing a soon-to-be-obsolete statement. A third is that most therapists and clients usually think in terms of alleviating pain, in terms of desensitization. I can also fall into these traps; however, when I am functioning at my best I think of the positive not just in terms of cognitions, but rather networks of associations, including thoughts and images that could be — but are not — connected to the target dysfunctional network. I also try not to forget that the effort of obtaining positive cognitions, even if they are superseded, may help awaken the information necessary for network integration to occur.

To briefly summarize my view:

1. The goal of EMDR is to encourage the integration of dysfunctional (negative) and functional (positive) associative networks, or schemas, thereby changing the dysfunctional network into a functional one.
2. The negative associative network may be conceptualized as the "problem." The positive material accessed or introduced may be referred to as the "solution."
3. As EMDR has been developed and taught, the positive cognition is the chief aspect of the positive network explicitly accessed before Category 3 activity begins.
4. When working with clients who have simple, straightforward problems, it is worthwhile for the therapist to conceptualize the positive cognition as part of a network or schema; however, it is most efficient and consistent with client goals to use the positive cognition as developed by Shapiro.
5. In working with clients who have more complex problems or impoverished positive schema, it is worthwhile to use a broader representation of the positive schema, and work with it more explicitly with the client.
6. The need for more elaborative work on the positive may not become apparent until Category 3 activity has been initiated.

Positive Schema

Definition and Conceptualization

Paralleling the earlier discussion of how thinking in terms of the AIP model may not affect the visible behavior of the therapist, thinking in terms of positive schema instead of positive cognitions will usually not affect the therapist's behavior in the assessment phase. Therefore, it is still most parsimonious to simply obtain a positive cognition and then proceed to the negative network (ask the client to return to imagining the visual image, ask about emotion, and so forth) to prepare the target associative network for Category 3 activity.

I realize that, in suggesting the broader conceptualization, I may be mucking up an easily understood, straightforward pattern of accessing. However, I think it is worth the risk to make the procedure more similar to what I am arguing is the underlying process in EMDR and psychotherapy in general: the integration of information that has been held in separate associative networks, not simply adding on a positive cognition. If this point of view is seen from the start, I think it less likely that EMDR will be mistaken for a simple desensitization technique, and that the therapist will be more effective and flexible in helping clients through difficult material.

There are three occasions prior to the beginning of the desensitization phase (the beginning of Category 3 activity) when it may be advisable to help the client access or form a fuller schema, adding elements such as visual images, ego ideals, and archetypes:

1. In the history and goal-setting activities of the first sessions when the client is identifying possible solutions to his negative associative networks and the strengths he brings to the endeavor.

2. When a client cannot accept the *possibility* of the positive cognitions discussed (a VoC of 1 suggests this). In this situation, which is fairly common for combat veterans, the positive schema may be introduced for discussion, then become an independent target for Category 3 activity. This process has recently been referred to in EMDR Institute training as *resource installation*.

3. When the client has a generally fragile adjustment with episodes of dissociation, especially when these episodes involve dangerous behavior. For these clients, considerable work in focusing on positive schema will be necessary before the trauma aspect networks are intentionally accessed.

    The positive cognition as part of a network containing many kinds of elements has already been discussed from a theoretical point of view. The original idea of expanding the positive cognition to the positive schema was not based on theory, but rather on observations of spontaneous "solutions" clients have developed in processing information, and therapist interventions (interweaves) made as processing was blocked. It is the incorporation of such clinical findings into a broader conceptualization of the process that makes fuller use of accelerated information processing.

    The clinical situation that I think of in reference to this idea is that of a client who saw a friend die near him in a battle. Intellectually, he knew he could not save him, yet he was overwhelmed by guilt for not having acted. This "survivor guilt," as it is often called, is a common phenomenon and is underrated as a source of distress. As the client did eye movement while recalling the episode, there was little change in his level of distress. I asked him where his friend is now. He said, "In heaven," and another set of eye movement proceeded. My client became calm and smiled. He said that he saw an image of his friend in heaven smiling at him. The positive information that began to connect with the associative network of the battle obviously contained more than just a positive self-statement. It also contained a visual image and a conceptualization of the "afterlife," as well as an emotional reaction. My client had accessed something more than a positive belief.

    Another, less dramatic, example occurred with a client who had been having problems at work, which he said pervaded his life to the extent that he was continually unhappy, no activity brought him pleasure. We targeted his work situation with EMDR, using conventional self-referent negative and positive cognitions, both in the initiation of the session and as interweaves when processing stalled; the client made no progress toward resolving his negative emotions. In the middle of the second session, as he followed his associations of gloom and despair, a pleasant picture of his granddaughter, smiling, occurred to him. This did not immediately result in complete resolution of his problems (which did improve markedly over the next few weeks), but it did bring him a moment of relief. The point is that the verbal material we had been accessing, such as the fact that there were many positive aspects to his life, including his family, had not brought him the relief that accompanied the image of his grandchild. Accessing the visual aspect of his positive network, the positive schema, seemed to provide the relief. It is my best guess that the extent to which the image of the granddaughter, perhaps representing an element of perspective, pervades the associative network that includes the work issue will determine how effective the intervention is.[11]

A simple example of a therapist-prompted schema occurred when a client was stuck in images of himself at age 9, being berated by adults over his failure to perform chores that were clearly beyond his ability. The client was asked to put an image of himself now, as an adult, in mind and have that adult image interact with the adults in his target image. He was an accomplished martial artist and constructed an image of himself in his martial arts uniform, going to the adults and telling them to leave the child alone. This produced considerable emotional relief.

Positive schema established at the beginning of treatment and cognitive interweave material have two similarities that warrant their being considered together. First, they have the same job in the proposed theoretical framework; to provide material to be combined with the negative network in order to create a reformulated adaptive network. Second, except in a few cases in which a paradoxical intervention[12] is initiated, the content of positive schema and interweaves is intended to be neutral ("It's over") or positive ("I learned from it"). They will, therefore, be discussed somewhat interchangeably. So an interweave described from a clinical setting may be suggested as a positive schema, material to access before Category 3 activity is initiated.

11. This is not to suggest that there weren't early life experiences and learned patterns of adjustment, in addition to current life difficulties, that still needed to be addressed for more complete resolution of the client's distress.
12. Paradoxical interventions must be used carefully; there has to be sufficient rapport that the client does not access so much negative material, such as the thought that the therapist is no longer an ally, that he quits the process. Let's say the client is himself a generally competent therapist who is working on troubling feelings and thoughts following the decompensation of a client, and is stuck on the notion that he didn't do a very good job and is therefore not competent. I might consider having the therapist make an exaggerated thought, such as "I am a horrible therapist" or "I am the worst therapist in the state," the target of Category 3 activity. Without sufficient rapport, the client may take the paradoxical intervention to be a statement of the therapist's view — thereby destroying the therapy.

It should also be pointed out that a paradoxical statement may access positive material in a variety of ways. Two possibilities are through evoking its contrast, as discussed earlier, and by accessing the idea that such ratings are absurd and not to be taken seriously.

Despite the obvious presence and value of the nonverbal aspects of positive schema, it is difficult to give them the prominence they deserve because it is so much easier to talk and write about the "head" than the "heart." I heard the comedian Emo Phillips make this point in a joke. In his sing-song, airy voice he said "The brain is the most interesting organ ... but then look what is telling me that."

The use of positive schema can be more involved than simple positive cognitions. If the therapist is first obtaining the negative and positive cognitions during the session in which Category 3 activity is to be initiated, there can be time problems with using positive schema. However, if the therapist begins to work on formulating the negative and positive aspects of the associative networks during the history and rapport-building session(s), then preparation for the Category 3 activity can go quickly in that session. In working with veterans with chronic combat-related PTSD, in many places in the DVA system it is both possible and clinically necessary, in most instances, to have several history/rapport-building/therapeutic contract sessions.

In some ways, broadly conceived positive schema is a vague area, where psychology, philosophy, and spirituality meet. For clients whose trauma challenges the basic assumptions that underlie the value of life, processing to resolution does not simply mean returning to the state one was in before the event. In these situations, areas that are often artificially kept separate during therapy fit together naturally and sometimes inescapably. From the psychological point of view, this is perhaps the place that humanistic[13] psychology is best integrated into EMDR. As Maslow (1968) pointed out, the traditional psychology of his time (and one which I am afraid may be becoming more firmly entrenched in clinical psychology) was one of deficits and disorders, insufficient to understand humanity. He wrote that a psychology of being and becoming, and ultimately transcendence, is necessary to comprehensively reflect humanity.

It has been a profoundly confusing, illuminating, and moving process for me to help search for positive cognitions and schema with clients who have been in war and witnessed themselves, their friends, and their beliefs destroy and be destroyed. My clients have sometimes killed those whom they were always taught to protect. They found themselves overwhelmed and helpless to act, or they acted in ways they later prayed they didn't, in situations they would feel impelled to have define the whole of their lives. They were effectively taught a set of combat values — which were often opposed to the spiritual or humanistic values by which they previously defined themselves — and then found themselves repeatedly in situations where one set of values or the other had to be violated. And there was no escape. Some of the people who lived through such situations have found ways to process those events; others have been effectively able to inhibit the

---

13. It may be interesting to consider that it is under the label *humanism*, a term of derision to many with strongly held religious beliefs, that spirituality may find a more scientifically acceptable way back into psychology.

accessing of the networks that include those events; some have come to me as clients to consult in this effort and have taught me enough to be of help to them.

In identifying (accessing) or constructing (introducing and accessing) positive schema, as with other aspects of therapy, the best place to start is by asking the client about the beliefs he has, in this case those that give him strength. (In taking history, I will have asked already about spiritual beliefs.) Clients will sometimes talk about their families, sometimes talk about living up to a standard they believe in, and sometimes talk about their spiritual beliefs. I may then go on to ask how these strength-giving forces interact with the target network. Often clients will say they do not relate to the target or that, when they think about the things that give them strength, they just end up feeling guilty. The therapist does not then try to convince the client to feel otherwise; he or she only raises questions and tries to find out what the client would like to have integrated into the target network. The goal is to help access or introduce the positive and to promote the client making connections with Category 3 activity.

Working with spiritual issues can be a delicate matter for a psychotherapist. Setting aside the acceptability of this subject to a radically scientific therapist, there are still the possible objections of the spiritually minded who may consider it blasphemous to employ spiritual beliefs as just another part of a class of potentially beneficial beliefs. (Fortunately, probably because of my limited social sphere, I have not yet run across this objection.) Because I recognize the power of spiritual beliefs to be, for some, the only avenue of relief from despair (James, 1902, 1958), I am especially careful to open the door to this area with focus on what the client (not I) thinks might be on the other side.

Earlier examples illustrated the basic concept of the positive schema; the following example, constructed from clinical experience, will illustrate the selection of the initial positive cognition, following the standard EMDR guidelines for positive cognitions, then introduce dialogue illustrating the development of a broader concept of the positive schema. I hope it is clear that the illustrations of establishing initial positive schema are equally applicable to interweave after processing has begun.

Start with the example of a combat veteran who participated with his comrades in bombarding an enemy village in which women, children, and old men were killed. (If he had initiated the activity without immediate provocation, the issues dealt with would be much more complex and involve the events leading up to this incident. For the sake of clarity, I will put the client in a more passive role and address the more difficult issue later.)

The initial target picture was of a child screaming; the negative cognition was "I'm a murderer."

THERAPIST: With this scene in mind, what words or belief would you prefer to have come to awareness?

CLIENT: I'd rather think it didn't happen.

THERAPIST: We both know we cannot change the past, but we can understand it, and ourselves, in ways that are less devastating. Even if you don't think it is completely true *now*, what belief would you prefer to have about yourself now, when you think about this episode?

CLIENT: I'd rather think that I'm basically a good person. But how could that be, if I did that?

THERAPIST: So, now thinking about that incident, at a gut level how believable is it to you, that phrase "I'm basically a good person"?

CLIENT: I don't believe it. Zero.

(Consistent with standard EMDR practice, this cognition, rated zero, is not accepted as the positive cognition.)

THERAPIST: I'm hearing you say that right now you can see no path to making peace with this event. What do your religious beliefs teach you about understanding this event in your life?

CLIENT: My religious beliefs didn't do me much good in 'Nam.

THERAPIST: So where do you stand now on that?

CLIENT: I still believe in God.

THERAPIST: What do your beliefs tell you about living with the things from Vietnam, how do you go on?

CLIENT: I don't think you can say it's OK to kill children.

THERAPIST: I don't know that much about your religion, but I do know that the concept of forgiveness probably wouldn't have been invented *if people were only forgiven when the action that needs forgiveness was completely OK in the first place.* So what are your beliefs about the path to forgiveness?

Forgiveness can be a highly complex issue. Processing of material may be blocked because there are strong alternative beliefs that, under the circumstances, the client did not do wrong; however, he believes he is supposed to think that he did. So the therapist's attempt to access forgiveness may be a mistake.

It should also be noted that a network containing guilt may have mistakenly required the belief that *because it occurred,* it was intended. This is a stance sometimes taken by people who dread loss of the sense of control more than having done wrong.

In the preceding and the next few interchanges, I am clearly and subtly accessing and/or introducing information. Usually it is in the form of questions, because I try to take the role of a fellow investigator, which is not difficult, because I truly am. I don't *know* the right answers. The times at which I introduce information, such as hypothesizing, that forgiveness would be unnecessary if it only applied to what was already acceptable, I try to do so tentatively. I also try to avoid being opinionless, as is seen in some Rogerian approaches, because to avoid expression of opinion is not consistent with the fact or impression of genuine human interaction, and I want my manner to continually stimulate client associative networks about the truth that he is dealing with a peer and an ally.[14]

> CLIENT: I guess I believe that you are forgiven if you repent, if you are sorry.
>
> THERAPIST: Then what happens?
>
> CLIENT: I guess you go on with your life.
>
> THERAPIST: Are you allowed to then find peace with your family?
>
> CLIENT: Yes.
>
> THERAPIST: So then, is there a thought or something that you would prefer to come to mind when this event is with you?
>
> CLIENT: I would like to think that forgiveness is possible.
>
> THERAPIST: Is there an image or picture that would go with that thought?
>
> CLIENT: I guess it could be a picture of me at peace.
>
> THERAPIST: Now as you think of the picture in the village, how believable is that thought, "Forgiveness is possible"?
>
> CLIENT: I still don't really believe it.
>
> THERAPIST: So what number on 1 to 7, with 1 as totally false at a gut level and 7 as complete belief?
>
> CLIENT: Maybe a 2.

14. I would likely be feeling considerable sadness and compassion myself, as I contemplated these events with my client. It is my best judgment that the client perceives this at some level, and it causes him to access helpful network material. If I could not feel compassion, then it is likely that unhelpful material would be accessed by the client. (I realize these are speculations.)

In this example, we have developed a new cognition about forgiveness, rather than self-evaluation as a good person. In the discussion of the path to peace, the client spontaneously brings up the issue of forgiveness, which I pursue because it is part of a possible clear path to processing. I introduce the idea of pairing an image with the cognition, even though I don't include it during the VoC rating; I have tried to help the client more fully access this aspect of his associative network around finding peace because it may make processing more likely. To more fully illustrate the many ways to access positive schema in the same situation, I will present an alternative dialogue:

THERAPIST: I'm hearing you say that right now you can see no path to making peace with this event. What do your religious beliefs teach you about understanding this event in your life?

CLIENT: I don't think you can forgive being part of killing children.

THERAPIST: It's kind of interesting how some of the most important, positive figures in history, including some saints, did some things in their early lives that anyone would regret. Let me ask you who is the most spiritually advanced or enlightened person you know or have ever heard of?

CLIENT: It is X. (X could be Malcolm X, Moses, Jesus, Buddha, or the client's grandmother — it can't matter to the therapist[15] who the figure is, only that the client see this person as part of the healing process.)

THERAPIST: Can you imagine how X might find peace with this event if he had been part of it? Can you imagine X talking to you? Please do that. (Pause) What might X say about the way to live with this?

CLIENT: I have to find a way to go on. I don't know. Maybe I can do good things in memory of those kids.

THERAPIST: With that target picture in mind, on a scale of 1 to 7...

Another spiritual path to promote processing in this client is one that I prefer.[16] As is possible with all the above suggestions, the following schema can be used as an interweave, to access or introduce, if there is no movement with earlier paths the client had taken:

15. When it does matter to the therapist who the figure is, he must be in a practice that is restricted to clients with similar beliefs.
16. My colleague Al Botkin has developed this approach differently and has used it very effectively with Karen Paddock in the context of a wonderfully supportive inpatient program.

THERAPIST: I'm hearing you say that right now you can see no path to making peace with this event. Let me ask you, what do you think happens to people after they die?

CLIENT: If they are lucky, they get buried.

THERAPIST: I mean, is there anything of them that lives on?

CLIENT: If they are good they go to heaven.

THERAPIST: Where do you think that child you see screaming is now?

CLIENT: In heaven, of course, of course.

THERAPIST: Can you imagine a picture of that? (Depending on a variety of factors, the therapist may also ask the client to say something in his mind to the child.)

CLIENT: Yes.

At this point in the work, if the client is emotionally moved, and depending on the time available, rapport, and other readiness and preparation factors, I would do Category 3 activity immediately; remember the work is to access and process. This is another way of saying: sometimes, don't stop for the VoC or to begin to focus the picture and negative cognition again. You can and must work with these elements later in order to process the whole associative network. Otherwise, the client is more likely to have a recurrence of his acute distress. Shapiro's protocol, ordering the accessing of information as she does, is very efficient and has proven to be successful; however, sometimes a different order is necessary or the best opportunity for the client to access and process the material will be lost.

The importance of later taking into account the aspects of the network avoided when one jumps into Category 3 activity is easily comprehended when one considers the beginning negative cognition, "I am a murderer." How this belief stands in the associative network must be assessed after there is some resolution of painful destructive emotion through processing the spiritual material. There may be more processing to do with this cognition or with other elements of the network, or the relief gained may be temporary.

But if, instead of saying "In heaven, of course, of course," the client says:

CLIENT: Yes, but what does that have to do with anything?

THERAPIST: Have you considered the possibility that you are the one holding on to that child's pain, not the child? Have you lived in a way you are proud of since the war?

CLIENT: No.

THERAPIST: Which do you think would be a better memorial for that child — your continuing to live like you have been, or doing positive things?

CLIENT: Doing positive things.

THERAPIST: So with the target picture in mind, how believable is the thought, "I can do positive things," on a scale of 1 to 7...

With such an intervention, clients sometimes see the victim as being at peace, and the negative network starts to resolve. Occasionally, a client will not be able to process his destructive negative material with verbal or imaginal work. In such a situation, the client may need to do something like volunteer work to meaningfully access, or create, the positive material necessary for him to process the target network. In this situation the positive schema would contain actual behavior. I should point out that a client's problems with avoidance do make this suggestion difficult to implement. Whether or not the client has had powerful guilt-producing trauma, he may be generally withdrawn and/or anhedonic. Before working with the associative networks that produced this mode of functioning, it may be necessary to simply access elements that contain positive activity (perhaps through guided imagery) and add Category 3 activity.

I have heard at least one person, aside from clients who believe they deserve to suffer, raise a moral question here, saying it is not desirable or appropriate for someone who has participated in the perpetration of trauma to be relieved of torment. In the most striking example, the person objecting was a noted PTSD psychotherapy researcher speaking at an international conference. There are several responses to this point that I find compelling. First, torment does not change the past, or make it less likely that horrible events will happen again, but it does increase the likelihood that the person in torment will not be able to function very well in accomplishing positive goals. Second, the role of psychotherapy is not to punish criminal or immoral behavior; the psychotherapist accepts the client to help him achieve acceptable goals. If the therapist does not believe the client's goals are prosocial, or at least socially neutral, then he should not accept the treatment contract. Third, especially in relationship to war, society as a whole contributes to that activity, so we may presume the therapist pays taxes, thereby supporting combat. From such a position, it is hypocritical for the therapist to judge the soldier as not deserving treatment.

Although I have not seen it happen, it occurred to me that it was possible that a client's religious beliefs could be disconfirmed by processing. At an EMDR conference in 1995, I had the opportunity to do a brief informal survey on this question. At a presentation conducted by Roger Solomon and Jeffrey Mitchell, the question of spirituality was raised. As an audience member, I asked if any other audience members had asked clients to focus on their spiritual beliefs and then do eye movements. About 20 people raised their hands. I asked then if any found their clients to disconfirm their religious beliefs. One person raised his hand and reported that the client in question was a minister. This survey was quite instructive on a number of levels, but for our purposes here it gives further reason to believe that spiritual interventions are likely to be helpful in processing.

In her book and her training workshops, Shapiro and her colleagues have offered a list of positive cognitions keyed to negative cognitions. That list is not intended to be complete or authoritative; rather, it is suggestive, as some of the cognitions may be counterproductive in some situations.[17] The list is only meant to stimulate the process of selection of cognitions when the client is bogged down. Similarly, I will be offering a companion list — extensively borrowed from a wide variety of sources, most of which have their roots in antiquity — of positive cognitions and possible accompanying noncognitive elements that may form schema, which (it is hypothesized) can unite with maladaptive associative networks formed around (often traumatic) events, to transform those networks to an adaptive state. In a sense these schema are possible "solutions" to the question, How does one live with these horrible events? The schema are divided into two categories: those that focus on people other than the client, and those that focus on the client and his self and world views. Clients who have been in combat or were otherwise involved in harm to others often have to progress through the first type of schema to get to the second.

These schema are introduced in the therapy session when the client needs them, either at the beginning of treatment or as treatment progresses, as illustrated in the foregoing dialogues. Out of this discussion, a simple positive cognition may develop. This does not mean, however, that we should consider the schema conceptualization irrelevant. As I see it, it is not only the positive cognition that influences the processing, but rather all of the material present in the discussion that contributes to the accessing of the positive, including — and this cannot be emphasized too strongly — what is accessed by the relationship with the therapist.

Developing Solutions

1. Solutions that first focus on people other than the client usually apply to situations in which the client feels guilt, often with grief as an underlying emotion. These solutions that allow the client to find peace often have the theme that, ultimately, good or innocence prevails. Specific examples of this type of solution follow:

Reward or relief comes to those who have suffered.   In the spiritual elaboration of this schema, the good and the innocent are rewarded in heaven

---

17. The positive cognition, "I am now in control," is especially likely to contain perfectionistic implications that can block complete processing. If a client chooses this one, among others, I am careful to explore that implication of perfection.

or through other spiritual effects, such as the accumulation of positive karma. Not only is their suffering temporary, but the negative experience leads to positive experience. In the clinical vignette above, the child who was killed is seen by the client as going to heaven. Expressed as the thought, "The child is in heaven," it is a positive cognition. Experienced with the notion of going on to a heavenly reward, with accompanying visual images, it becomes a schema. The image of going to heaven is only one of many possible solutions to a negative network that contains suffering and death.

As mentioned, my colleague Al Botkin has developed a similar approach. My interpretation of Botkin's method is that, after doing preliminary work, he invites the client to be aware of the connection with the person who died, and then do a set of eye movements. What follows depends on the client's response. Botkin reports that clients usually have spontaneously positive images of the deceased, and achieve powerful and lasting forgiveness and resolution with this approach to grief. It should be pointed out, however, that this intervention takes place within the context of an intensive 5-week inpatient program, as where a small group of clients and therapists establish relationships that access powerful elements of safety, acceptance, and expectation of positive treatment effects. And this program is embedded in another supportive PTSD treatment program, directed by Orv Lips.

The memory of friends who have died is better honored by living a positive life than by prolonging suffering. The client can be asked if this is so, following a discussion of the friends and their positive qualities. The client can be asked to evoke images of the friends speaking to him, followed by Category 3 activity. (This is further elaborated in Chapter 5.)

The victim's suffering is complete and the pain now is held only by the client. The client is then responsible for the release of the victim's pain, because the victim has already released as much he or she can.

Continued suffering for the victims adds to the amount of pain in the world, as do other self-destructive acts, such as suicide, and prevents good, which the client cannot promote if he is suffering debilitating pain. To illustrate this point, I often tell my clients a story that Francine Shapiro offers: a person sought out a famous writer and said he would like to do something for him to pay him back for the pleasure his books had brought. The writer said, "You don't get it; you don't pay back, you pay forward." In a situation like the one described here, I will sometimes tell this story and then initiate eye movement.

Failure to find comfort or maintain self-respect negates efforts to comfort or value others. A client who had financial ups and downs had to rely on assistance from his brother when he had some business problems. Among other difficulties, he was depressed, which he attributed to this dependency, even though he knew it to be temporary. After several sets of eye movements, he recalled how vulnerable some civilians he helped in Vietnam had seemed, and he believed that, if he didn't always do his share, he would be vulnerable like the Vietnamese. I asked him if he respected the Vietnamese even though they needed his help. He replied, with certainty, that he did. I then asked: What does it say about the sincerity of your respect for the Vietnamese if you cannot respect yourself when you accept help? He smiled and said he hadn't thought of that before. I then asked him to do a set of EM. The tension he had felt previously was completely resolved.

This same principle can be accessed in a Gestalt-like interweave by having the client carry on an imaginary conversation or a role-playing conversation with the therapist.

There is a fundamental relationship among people that transcends even the most painful experiences.   Most religions have their own versions of this theme, often associated with Asian philosophies. Additionally, one can imagine a "nonreligious" spiritual image in which the life force of the grieved person radiantly explodes, joining with the life force of the universe. William James (1901) notes in *The Varieties of Religious Experience* that, across most known religions, the mystical state of grace includes the expansion of awareness and the unity of all.

2. Solutions that first focus on the client's ability to transform himself, his self-concept, and/or his recognition of his situation are generally based on the underlying notions that life is, or at least has the potential to be, progressive and that meaning can be created. Just as good can win out in the attainment of final reward (as discussed in the schemas above), good can be made from bad for the client. Human beings have the power to improve and progress. The schema discussed here concern a client's pain related to beliefs about himself and the nature of the world, rather than about the suffering that comes from empathy or sympathy for others. Solutions can range from basic cognitions, such as "I am safe now" or "It's over" to elaborate schema containing images of family members or historical figures providing comfort or wisdom.

When using schema in this category, I find it helpful to remind clients that the painful memory they are accessing exists only as a network of chemical and electrical relationships that has not received the message that the event is over, that it is in the past. I acknowledge that this is a very powerful network that contains much pain, but remind them that they have the ability to make new chemical and electrical connections.

Schema in this category may be spiritual or not. The possibility of expiation of sins (real or imagined) and spiritual redemption for the client are in this category. The notion of progress, that we have an innate propensity to learn from or build on previous problems or mistakes, is a powerful secular version of this. This solution, which contains positive cognitions such as "I can learn from this" or "I can use this to do better in the future," has a strong modern base in the humanistic psychology of Maslow (1970), whose hierarchy of needs describes people as having (if not blocked) the innate tendency to move toward self-actualization.

Knowledge of the client's history and espoused values are particularly important when helping a client develop positive schema.

Bringing in a third party. In elaborating a schema, images of others can be helpful. Images of beloved or admired people may be evoked. The client might be asked to imagine what one of these figures might provide as a positive cognition. Discussion of respected ancestors and the struggles and mistakes they might have made and overcome can be useful in accessing the notion that we can overcome difficulties or learn from mistakes. I find it helpful, on occasion, to do Gestalt therapy type work to access images and thoughts of a loved and loving grandparent who can engage the client in "conversation" that may lead to promotion of a progress schema.

The third party can even be the client himself, going back in imagination to lend support to the younger version of himself. This is sometimes referred to as "inner child work" (see Price, 1996, for discussion). One client worked on a still-troubling situation from childhood when she was walking across a narrow bridge on a camping trip with a friend's family. She got halfway across, was terrified and couldn't move. She was left behind for a few minutes and, when the family returned for her, she was simply encouraged to proceed. As she spoke between sets of eye movements, she was obviously partially reexperiencing the event. I asked her if she could imagine someone coming to get her and help her across. She imagined the friend's brother doing so and did another set of EM, but was still obviously upset. I asked her who she wanted to come help her. She said she wanted to help herself. I asked her to imagine this and she did EM. This resulted in the resolution of her anxiety.

For this client, the image of helping herself was the schema version of cognitions such as "It's in the past," " I was a little girl then and am an adult now and can handle situations like that," or "I can help myself." Again, the positive schema was introduced as interweave; however, it could just as easily have been presented in the place of a positive cognition in the course of EMDR treatment.

Clients who are not suffering because of actions they regret, but are bothered and discouraged by slow movement toward their goals or by external attack, may be helped by recalling events and stories of persistence being rewarded. Some examples might be Frederick Douglass or Helen Keller. Spiritual versions likewise abound in most of the world's most widely followed religions. The stories of Jesus, Buddha, and Mohammed are stories of defeat or suffering that lead to wondrous outcomes. Needless to say, the therapist must be careful in addressing spiritual beliefs, as each client may have a different interpretation of Scripture, or even doubts about the therapist having the standing to address these beliefs.

People create the meaning of events and themselves. This is the basis of the existential position, perhaps most movingly described by Victor Frankl (1946, 1959). If the death or loss of another leads us to define life as futile and full of meaningless pain, then that is what life is. But if we use loss to inspire us to recognize our power to create happiness and limit pain, then that is what life is.

On occasion, with a client who is unable to find other solutions, who is in great despair, I have brought in the example of Winston Smith from Orwell's *1984* (1949). Many clients are familiar with either the book or the movie, and I initiate discussion by reminding them of how Winston Smith, under the threat of torture, betrayed his girlfriend to the agents of Big Brother. I tell them that I think the universal emotional power of the work comes from Orwell's illustration that each of us has a weak point that can be used to make us do almost anything. If we accept this — whether one has actually committed transgression or not — we accept that we are capable of it, and this knowledge can lead to despair. We may then cope with an event or knowledge of our potential by trying to make ourselves so strong that nothing can ever lead to our transgressing, or transgressing again. However, simply making ourselves stronger is not a good solution, because we never can be absolutely sure of our strength. At the end, Smith walks by his girlfriend, who has been released, as has Smith, because they are no longer dangerous to the state; they have given in to despair. Their problem is not their weakness to threats of torture, but rather giving up afterward, letting the vulnerability define them. I explain that this is the problem for all of us, more painful and immediate for those who have faced extreme conditions, such as combat, but still the problem for all of us. However, we can find peace with our weakness, many have done it before, and this can be our true strength.[18]

Once again, interweaves such as the one based on *1984* depend upon the therapist's willingness to discuss this kind of depth of despair. The manner in which the therapist broaches the issue will likely access as much or more curative material as the content of the interweave.

There are many metaphors and symbols that can be created and employed from the basic position that we create our own meaning. It must be noted that the following schema are not exclusive, and that one that is effective for one client may be counterproductive for another.

Life is a journey or exploration.   The client may envision himself journeying on a path through a variety of terrains and challenges. One client, an industrial salesman with unsupportive boss and family members, was subject to frequent anxiety and panic attacks as well as a generally ego-dystonic, pugnacious attitude. He found the suggestion to consider life a journey that had some battles, rather than a battle that had some journeying in it, when paired with EM, to reduce his anxiety level and to be helpful in maintaining this reduction as new challenges came up.

Another path toward this schema has been helpful to clients with good imaginative ability who have not been able to accept the possibility of

18. The serenity prayer addresses this point quite effectively.

emotional resolution. I asked a client to imagine a spaceship landing and friendly aliens asking her to take a journey through the outer reaches of the universe, exploring the stars, planets, and various life forms, including even time travel. She imagined this briefly; then I asked, "If this happened, how would your past be with you, could you make peace with it?" The answer was "yes." I then asked the client to participate in EM. We then engaged in discussion of positive schema and established one for her.

Engagement in struggle is part of the definition of life. Illustrating this point and the point that one person's problem is another's solution, another client demonstrated the value in some situations of seeing oneself as a battler. This client, a mechanical engineer, had severe financial pressures, marital problems, medical problems, and a history of being abused as a child. His initial goal was to improve his social and employment relationships, necessary to maintain a platform for working on the other problems. He succeeded in this area by targeting, in therapy, work with a related childhood incident. However, he found himself extremely discouraged when he decided to take on limiting smoking, which was essential to help control an acute health problem. When we targeted specific situations in which he could change this behavior, he became even more discouraged, saying that he didn't know if he could deal with any more problems. He felt like he was fighting off too many things. I reminded him how well he had done with some of the issues we had already worked on and asked him to consider these problems as opponents he was fighting, and to visualize an image of this. He brought forward an image of tigers attacking him. I asked him to consider fighting these tigers one at a time. He imagined this and did some EM. After the first set, he said that he felt good about defeating the first tigers, but that the next one might beat him. We continued EM with this image. He next reported that he was fighting the tiger mightily, and he was no longer discouraged. In subsequent sessions, this client reported significant improvement in limiting his smoking.

Meaning does not have to be tied to self-judgment. Schema in this group attack the notion of self-judgment as tied to specific activities or the validity of self-judgment at all. Separating evaluation of the self from specific event is at least as old as the idea "Hate the sin, love the sinner." I often borrow ways of conveying this from the work of other therapists.

"Dis-identification." Roberto Assagioli (1965) describes the essential processes of "dis-identification" as helping the client discontinue identifying the self as identical with a specific element, such as a current feeling or thought. In a novel way of implementing this idea, Steven Hayes (1987) asks the client to consider the content of awareness as a game among many competing ideas and feelings. In a given situation we might be afraid, angry, and curious, all at the same time and have simultaneous thoughts of running, fighting, or watching. These various elements "fight it out" and action is

determined by which side wins. Likewise, self-judgments may be in conflict. For simplicity's sake, let's take an example of a two-sided conflict, such as the decision between whether we are basically a strong or weak person. We may consider this a chess game with moves by black pieces representing one side and white pieces representing the other. The question for the client then is: If the pieces represent evidence for one side or the other in this battle, what represents the self? Most clients do not guess the answer, which is "the board" (p. 360). Hayes points out to clients that it is part of our nature to have all kinds of thoughts and feelings; these lead to positive and negative experiences and everything in between. However, what causes us sustained unhappiness is when we forget that the self is not these specific elements, but rather it is enduring and transcends the specific. The discussion of this concept can lead clients to positive schema that do not refute specific negative judgments, but rather diminish the strength of the concept of *self-judgment*. For clients who cannot restrain from being judgmental, it at least allows them to judge by potential rather than by past actions.

"I accept myself deeply and completely, even though I still have this problem." Roger Callahan (1994) in his early work sometimes had clients repeat this statement, derived from Carl Rogers (Callahan, 1994a), while they tapped themselves on the edge of the hand. Callahan had clients do this when desensitization was blocked. Although he minimized the value of the statement itself and believes that the hand-tapping provides the major effect, I have sometimes found this to be an effective positive schema when paired with any Category 3 activity.

The notion of self-acceptance can be tied to a Darwinian perspective, specifically when helping clients accept "unacceptable" thoughts or feelings that come up during trauma. Thoughts such as "I'm glad it wasn't me" when a friend is killed nearby, or fascination or even excitement when witnessing or participating in horrible events. It can be helpful to speculate with the client how these kinds of responses might be adaptive for the survival of the species and how the client himself had learned to adapt. For example, interest in or excitement at observing horrible events could have led our ancestors to acquire useful information needed for survival or to suppress accompanying panic that would lead to destruction. People who had these kinds of responses survived to pass them on to offspring — those who didn't, didn't survive. The client then may be helped to see these responses as unavoidable, as an acceptable part of his nature.

In this context it might also be helpful to discuss Karl Jung's understanding of human nature, how a wide variety of impulses and needs are deeply ingrained, and how it is likely some may present persistently and destructively if they are not accepted in positive, if limited, form.

Who's the judge? Sometimes clients report low self-esteem as their problem and include this as a negative cognition in a form similar to "I am worthless." I find it sad and ironic when low self-esteem is explicitly stated, because it seems likely that they came to this conclusion with the "help" of someone who, in the interest of mental health, encouraged the expansion of some specific negative thought or situation into this more inclusive and depressing concept. Usually the client has heard the suggestion that he work on having higher self-esteem, and sometimes the suggestion even includes a specific reason for the client to have this elevated esteem. When the client complains of low self-esteem, I sometimes find it helpful to ask them to expand on the idea and ask if this means they do not respect themselves and their opinions. They usually answer "yes."

> THERAPIST: We both recognize that you are here seeking my help because I am an authority on psychology, on understanding people. I have a Ph.D. and years of experience in this area. (I will often mention some of my specific accomplishments, laying it on thick.) Now, let's say I think you are a decent person, and very worthy. And that you are capable of making good decisions. Basically, I disagree with your view of yourself. If your problem is low self-esteem, I declare you cured.

> CLIENT: No. I don't think you can judge me like that.

> THERAPIST: What? If you are worthless and do not esteem yourself, how is it that you can disagree with me about a matter in which I am an expert?

At this point, clients sometimes laugh, and I make it explicit that universal negative self-judgments are not particularly accurate or useful. If this intervention is used because the client was having difficulty with the positive cognitions stage at the beginning of therapy, I then go on to ask again about positive cognitions. If this intervention is used as an interweave, I would ask the client to resume Category 3 activity after the discussion. Even when the discussion produces just a positive cognition, I see it as having accessed a whole positive network that may increase the probability of integrating positive information into the target network.

Meaning changes depending on perspective. Vietnam veterans in particular, because of what they learned about the politics of the war during or after their service, and how the war ended, believe they fought for "nothing" and that a friend died for "nothing." (Several veterans have told me of how televiewing the fall of the U.S. Embassy was personally disastrous for them.) The accompanying emotion is anger at the "forces" responsible for the loss of the war, rendering the loss of life meaningless.

There are two different perspectives that I usually choose. One is asking the client to consider that he (or his friend) went to battle for his own reasons, and I ask the client to provide these. If "patriotism" or "doing the right thing" isn't mentioned, I'll ask if that is part of it. Very few clients do not endorse this positive cognition. I then ask if you couldn't just as accurately say that he (or his friend) went to battle because he thought it was right, and somebody else's view or purposes can never change that. I then ask the client to imagine what he would have had to do to avoid the war and to imagine how he would be now if he had done that. Very few can even imagine having avoided it. Accessing memories of themselves making choices, and of their families at the time of the war, can be a powerful way of bringing forth information that will help process this kind of "fought/died for nothing" associative network. It is also helpful to remind the client that recognizing that his, or his friend's, decision had something to do with the death may be a way of honoring and respecting the friend or the client's younger self.

The second type of perspective is that of time. I initiate a discussion of politics since the war, and ask the client to consider how the war in Vietnam, with its drain on Soviet resources, and the license it may have given the Soviets to invade Afghanistan, may have led to the fall of that power, and, thus, the potential for freedom in the former Eastern Bloc. Of course I recognize how this change may have made some things worse in various ways, but the point still stands that the sacrifice in Vietnam — despite the motives and plans of the politicians — may have long-term benefit. I then may remind the client that he is basing feelings on an understanding frozen in time, frozen at the time of the incident, or at the time of the collapse of the embassy. I may ask if there is another equally accurate way to understand events so that there isn't more pain attached than is needed. Depending on the situation we may then talk some more or do Category 3 activity.

In this context I like to repeat the ancient story of the Chinese farmer whose horse ran away; I first read it in one of Alan Watts' (1975) books. The story continues:

> ...that evening the neighbors gathered to commiserate with him since this was such bad luck. He said "May be." The next day the horse returned, but brought with it six wild horses, and the neighbors came exclaiming at his good fortune. He said, "May be." And then, the following day, his son tried to saddle and ride one of the wild horses, was thrown and broke his leg. Again the neighbors came to offer their sympathy for the misfortune. He said, "May be." The day after that, conscription officers came to the village to seize young men for the army, but because of the broken leg the farmer's son was rejected. When the neighbors came in to say how fortunate everything had turned out, he said "May be." (p. 31)

The story best illustrates one of the most important points of this section for those who have become committed to painful judgments about themselves and life: uncertainty about the meaning of events — besides more accurately reflecting life — also brings some relief. An ancillary point that may benefit the many clients who are withdrawn and feel uncomfortable with much conversation is that you don't have to talk much to have a lot of concerned friends.

Life is short.   Veterans with chronic suicidal ideation often have difficulty coming up with any positive cognition or schema; they have not acted on the belief that suicide is a good answer, but they are tempted. Life seems long and gruesome. In this situation, offering positive cognitions or schema may be taken by the client to represent lack of understanding by the therapist and break rapport. I have asked some veterans to think back upon their early lives, to incidents of childhood, and then asked them to consider how long ago it feels like; then, project themselves into the future, imagining themselves living a long life, and from that position looking back at how long life felt. Several clients have found this perspective comforting for themselves, and also in contemplating the shortened lives of others.

> CLIENT: My life is miserable, I don't see the sense in going on. It's wrong to kill myself but I just don't see the sense to it. It just drags on and on.
>
> THERAPIST: Think back to your childhood; do you remember any events clearly?
>
> CLIENT: Yeah, I remember when I got lost in third grade. It feels like yesterday.
>
> THERAPIST: What was that — 35, 40 years ago?
>
> CLIENT: Yeah.
>
> THERAPIST: It feels like yesterday?
>
> CLIENT: Yeah.
>
> THERAPIST: Let's say, just for discussion's sake, you live to 80 or 90. Then, looking back to now, will it feel like yesterday?
>
> CLIENT: Yeah, I guess.
>
> THERAPIST: Life is short, we get a blink or two in eternity, some of us get more, some less. We make what we can of it. Can we do some eye movement?

Concluding Comments

This chapter has been an elaboration of the concept of the negative and positive cognitions in EMDR. As these concepts are introduced by Shapiro, they are set parts of a standard (in the sense of structured, not, unfortunately, in the sense of universally used) psychotherapy method. I have attempted to use some of my clinical experience to add to the understanding of the cognition in psychotherapy. Remember that it is difficult to know the contribution of the content of the cognitive component to successful processing. It may be that the therapist has helped the client by eliciting or introducing cognitive content, or it may be that in the process of coming up with cognitive material, other material has been accessed or introduced that allows for complete processing. For example, the therapist's allusion to literature, such as *1984*, may stimulate the belief that the therapist is a truly clever fellow and, if such a clever fellow is interested in the client, that evokes other positive material that allows for continued processing.

chapter 5

Category 3 Activity and Its Vicissitudes

Desensitization: Beginning, Preparation, and Mechanics

Shapiro refers to this next stage, where Category 3 activity is initiated, as "desensitization," which is consistent with her initial focus on resolving the negative aspect of the experience. In later conceptualizations, this stage of treatment was considered the time when desensitization occurred as a byproduct of reprocessing.[1] In its simplest form, the desensitization stage consists of guiding the client in successive sets of eye movement, during which there is psychological movement, until processing is complete. Henceforth, *movement* will refer to the continuation of processing; that is, some aspect of the experience is changing in a noncircular manner. Clients are told in EMDR directions that this might be emotions, body sensation, thoughts, or any other aspects of experience. Movement may be immediately experienced by the client either as positive or negative, pleasant or painful.

There are some clinical observations I think are worth sharing here. In the preparation stage, when clients are informed of their control of the procedure, I am careful to emphasize that the client can ask me to continue eye movement — just as he can have me stop. Sometimes clients have to be reminded of this: I have stopped EM, noticed the client was still actively processing, asked the client if he wanted to continue, and on that instruction resumed the set of EM.

The decision about which Category 3 activity to offer the client is a matter not yet experimentally resolved. I recommend starting with eye movement because of the amount of clinical experience supporting it, the feedback available to the therapist from the client's tracking, the ease in automating the stimulus, and because it avoids any potential problems of physical contact between the therapist and client. When eye movement is first demonstrated

---

1. On the way to complete processing there may be some periods where clients do not feel discomfort around a target event; however, more complete accessing (sometimes occurring naturally, as an anniversary date) may demonstrate that only partial desensitization has occurred.

with the client, it is vital to establish a distance the client finds comfortable. I do not negotiate rate, direction, or width at that time; I think these discussions distract from the process and, when negotiated outside the actual desensitization stage, do not perform well in actual use.[2] It is a good idea to let clients know in advance that while they are doing the eye movements you might make encouraging comments or need to give verbal prompts.

If clients complain about the rate or width of movement, I quickly change to conform to their wishes. Sometimes clients say "I'm not doing it right." I will often ask them to start with that and then initiate another set of eye movements. (I note to myself that this may be reflecting a self-schema of incompetence or, alternatively, a habit of *reporting* incompetence even though it is not strongly believed.) However, to maintain rapport it is sometimes necessary to make a supportive comment about how he or she is doing it correctly (which may access positive emotions, and perhaps a thought that the therapist is concerned about the client's well-being) before reinitiating eye movement. Response to persistent problems will be discussed below.

When there is a break in the processing, divergent from following the client experience or therapist-directed focusing, such as someone ignoring the "do not disturb" sign and knocking at the door, I find the best way to resume with minimal distraction is to ask the client to begin by being aware of any discomfort that remains, then lead another set of EM. If the client says there is no discomfort, consider asking him to bring back the original target scene and reevaluate for successful processing.

I rarely begin with the prescribed 25 back-and-forth movements; I usually begin with at least 50. I wish I had some empirical support for this but, alas, I think it comes from the primitive notion that if a little is good, a lot must be better. This does bring up the question of when to stop. There is no clear way of knowing this, but there are some strong, clinically supported guidelines of when *not* to stop. First, if the client's eyes stop following the therapist, or slow down spontaneously, *do not* stop then. If the eyes slow down, slow down the stimulus movements with them, and verbally encourage the client to keep moving. If the client's eyes stop altogether, and he is not obviously stopping because he wants to chat, it is essential to get his eyes moving again. Wave your hand in a nonthreatening way, give simple instructions, gradually increase the volume as you speak. There is a good chance your client is beginning to dissociate and you should help him attend again to his surroundings. I usually do this by calling his name and asking simple questions orienting him to his surroundings.

When the client begins to show emotion, continue eye movement until the emotion starts to abate. This may be several minutes or more. Simultaneously, make gentle supportive comments. Shapiro suggests choosing a metaphor during the preparation stage for use at these times. It is tempting to say something like "good, keep going" to a client who is strongly emoting.

2. As with other technique preferences, therapists are advised to not follow my suggestions if they disagree — clients can often perceive when something is offered without confidence and this sometimes accesses material that can prevent further processing.

I think there are potential problems for abuse victims who were told they were being "good" when they were abused, or for clients who are sensitive to external evaluation; however, my clients usually report that my comments helped but they don't remember exactly what was said. I prefer to say something supportive yet neutral that reinforces acknowledgment of the events. This includes such comments as " Just notice it" or "Let yourself (or your brain) sort it out." For clients who seem on the verge of being overwhelmed and need to be comforted, especially childhood sexual abuse victims, Shapiro has recommended stronger comments, closer to positive cognitions, such as "It's over now."[3] The comments made should fit with the known history.

On rare occasions (I think I know of three), clients leave their seats and partially relive the trauma. If the client is continuing — or can be quickly encouraged to continue — EM, then the therapist should continue. If the EM have stopped, the therapist then must work to reorient the client.

Most of the time strong emotion (crying, heavy breathing) is not shown; at these times, the length of a set of Category 3 activity can be based on a routine number of repetitions. Sometimes clients delay their breathing, and I wait until they exhale before I stop. Similar principles can be used with electric lights, hand tapping, and auditory stimulation. When using eye movements I typically change directions every few sets, unless the client rejects the change. I'll say something to the effect, "Let's try this direction," and begin diagonal or infinity symbol patterns. Shapiro has recommended directional change when there is no movement in the content of client consciousness or, if the client reports a headache, directional change may prevent the blocking of movement, or allow for the discovery of a preferred movement direction. With tactile stimulation, I sometimes change rhythm. The inclusion of regular changes in movement is also based on the untested theoretical notion that in some cases processing may stop because of habituation to the stimulus (failure of the orienting response?).

When a set of eye movements ends, standard instructions include "Rest/let it go/blank it out, and take a deep breath." However, some flexibility in wording may be desirable. Early in my use of EMDR, it was clear that some clients found "letting it go" and "blanking out" difficult and disruptive to progress since they couldn't do either. Consequently, when a set of eye movement is complete I simply ask the client to take a deep breath (I also take a deep breath) and, after a pause, ask the client "What comes to awareness now?" After working with the client for a while, I usually don't even ask for the deep breath. Clients do it spontaneously.

Clients sometimes say everything that occurred to them, with considerable elaboration, during the whole eye movement period. It is important, at first, to listen attentively without interruption; however, if it appears that the client believes he is supposed to do this or is using the elaboration to avoid, I sometimes tell him it is most important to know what was going on when

---

3. Shapiro advises using the interweave principles of safety, responsibility, and choices in making supportive comments.

the eye movement stopped. Clients also sometimes talk as they are process-ing. Initially, I believed that this did not hurt processing. Experience and conversations with other practitioners have confirmed that the client provid-ing a running narrative is not disruptive while strong emotion is being shown. However, if the narrative does not accompany emotion, clients seem to proc-ess more effectively when they are asked to wait to talk until later. I may explain that I think talking during eye movements makes it more difficult for the client to attend nonverbal aspects of the process. When presented this way, I have not yet found the request to delay talking to break rapport.

The wording one uses to initiate a next set of eye movements may be important. I prefer, when beginning a set of eye movements immediately after a client's report, to say "Begin with that." I will add "and notice what happens" for clients who tend to get stuck, or believe that they are supposed to stay focused on the target, sometimes adding prompts, such as "Notice whatever you get — pictures, thoughts, emotions, feelings, just notice what happens." Even though clients are given clear instructions before Category 3 activity begins, it is often difficult to remember that one is not supposed to stay focused on the target event, but rather "let whatever happens happen." The difficulty therapists have in correctly following this instruction under-scores the difficulty clients are likely to have.

Sometimes clients report that they have been counting the eye movements instead of focusing on other content of consciousness. As always, they can be asked to begin with that. Some of my colleagues have suggested longer sets of eye movements when this occurs. Alternatively, the client may be reassured that this is all right, to just notice what happens. In this situation shorter sets of eye movements might be tried with some direction back to an aspect of the target network. Marcia Whisman (personal communication, Sept. 1997) discusses the counting as a way of ritualizing for obsessive-compulsive clients, and has recommended a number of disruption strategies, including increased verbal contact during processing.

I have found it advantageous to use a stick or light bar[4] rather than my fingers to guide eye movement. The vast majority of clients are not bothered by the use of an EMDR "aid" and I have found it necessary to prevent arm discomfort. Following the lead of my colleague Jim Moore, I use half of an arrow, the feather half. The one I use was made by a Native American craftsman, and some of my clients find it a positive symbol. When holding the arrow I keep my thumb on the top so that I can use the wrist, elbow, and shoulder joints, either individually or in combination, to provide the movement. Varying the movement can reduce fatigue. Of course, I am describing my own experience and make no claim for expert medical or kinesiological knowledge in providing this example. More recently, I have found that at least 75% of my clients prefer the light bar. They report it is easier to follow.

4. A light bar is an electronic device. In consists of a strip of small light bulbs arranged in a row that direct the client's eyes in the direction and speed desired.

When Movement Stops: Sample Dialogues

Shapiro makes extensive recommendations, in her book and in EMDR training, about actions to take when movement stops. I will repeat her comments as little as possible, but sometimes the basics must be mentioned. My goal is to add to her suggestions, provide additional clinical examples, and place her recommendations in the context of the four-activity model.

"It Doesn't Work"

I judge that processing has stopped in three situations, discussed in the following sections.

The client continues to insist, often from the second set of eye movements, that "it" is not working, often accompanied by comments that he is doing it wrong or a variation of this theme.

This response may reflect the client's ambivalence concerning change, which is an extension of a general schema of inadequacy or incompetence. The first thing to do is ask the client to "Start with that":

CLIENT: I'm not doing it right. Nothing is happening.

THERAPIST: Start with that. (*Continue EM*)

CLIENT: I'm not moving my eyes correctly. I know I'm just too tough a case.

If this point is reached, continued attempts at Category 3 activity will not often be successful. If the therapist deems rapport to be in danger if Category 3 activity continues or if he makes direct attempts to convince the client to proceed, then I recommend going back to the instructional phase, in which the theory of treatment is explained and more positive elements are accessed. Stopping the "scheduled activity" and returning to an earlier stage may access associative networks in which the client has more comfortable emotions that go along with perceiving the control he actually has, and new material that may be necessary for processing is introduced.

I have done this with diagrams, which I call, with no particular claim to originality, maps of the networks. Most recently, these maps begin with writing down the contents of the mind/brain that we have been first targeting, delineating the specific elements — the visual image, thoughts, feelings, sensations — and clarifying that these are connected, which I illustrate by drawing lines connecting them and a circle around them. Scattered around the page, I then add other specific elements, both negative (of the painful emotional events) and positive (beliefs and images). Drawing a larger "circle," now including one of the new elements, I further explain how the "solutions" are not fully enough connected to the target network, and that the EM expands the area of connection, leading to a more optimal level of existing connections. (I will include a discussion of declarative and nondeclarative memory processing when appropriate). By drawing other, increasingly expanded, enclosures[5] I show how the direction in which the area of connection expands can be influenced, but not controlled, by the therapist, through a variety of Category 1 and 2 interventions.

As an example, consider a client whose therapeutic goal is to overcome anxiety related to his supervisor at work. Even though he has generally done well and had good performance reviews from this supervisor in the past, the supervisor, as he has done to all the employees, has called him incompetent and publicly criticized him. The client also reports a history of getting poor grades in school, even though he gives every indication of having had sufficient aptitude to do well. He has memories of other kids making fun of him and of a teacher and his father criticizing him for his stupidity. Obviously, even with this little history there are rich veins that therapists of many orientations might explore, but for simplicity's sake and following the principle of recognizing the client's right to set goals, we will begin with this example on the face of it.

The first stage of a map for a client includes the elements the client has identified in the "assessment" stage of the standard EMDR protocol. Lines among the negative elements are drawn quickly and sketchily, and the circle is drawn around the negative elements, with the positive element excluded. As I refer the client to our earlier conversations, I write other elements, negative and positive, hidden and known, explaining how the solutions are blocked off and not connected because the connecting process can be painful. I explain how the mind/brain defends against the inclusion process at the same time it invites it. After adding the new elements, I draw a couple of different enclosures showing how, when the connection process begins, it may begin with positive, soothing inclusions, or it may begin with more painful material. But if the process is allowed to continue, my experience is that the "solution" does get included and there is completion of processing, which means the digesting out of maladaptive negative emotions and often the conversion of sensory stimuli to simple knowledge that an activity occurred.

In the context of this explanation, the client's resistive statement can be added, and graphically be considered by the client as another element that is part of the negative associative network, there to prevent the pain of doing the connection work. It should also be mentioned that sometimes this kind of map may be used for clients before they get stuck. It can be especially helpful if the therapist believes the quicker explanations are not clear.

If this does not succeed in improving adaptive processing, consider the suggestions listed for the next two types of problems.

No Change
The client reports that all aspects of the experience during the previous set of Category 3 activity remain unchanged, without volunteering pessimistic comments about the procedure.

5. Yes, it gets messy, but that doesn't interfere. Also the map is only two-dimensional and the mental associations are of vast dimensions, so I don't make much of an attempt to place elements in proximity on any one dimension. The attempt to make hierarchical maps, such as Chemtob et al. (1988), is admirable but can be misleading.

When this occurs, the therapist has choices from three categories of intervention. He can help the client access a different aspect of already stored information, introduce new information, or change Category 3 activity. Following Shapiro, when working with failure to change, it is most efficient to change Category 3 activity, increase the number of eye movements, change direction, and/or change the type of activity, going from eye movement to hand tapping, for example. When Category 3 changes do not succeed in promoting processing, simply directing the client to the associative network's specific aspects — visual image, sounds, feelings — often facilitates processing. When neither Category 3 changes nor accessing activities produce movement, then consider the suggestions for the next type of problem.

Change Leads Nowhere

Aspects of the experience continue to change, but lead back to the same point, with no reduction in distress. The therapist must help the client access a different aspect of his associative networks or introduce new information. Deciding which of many possible interventions to make at this point is a clinical decision, based on the therapist's assessment of the client's situation.

My recommendation for a first intervention is to explicitly consider the notion that the therapeutic intervention is a partnership and simply ask the client what he believes might be preventing further processing. (This is among the simplest of what Shapiro refers to as cognitive interweaves.) I listen to the client's response, then generally follow with Category 3 activity.

THERAPIST: So what do you think has you stuck?

CLIENT: If I keep thinking about this, I might cry and I don't want to.

THERAPIST: OK, start with that. (*Proceed with a set of EM*)

Another simple approach is to ask the client to imagine the worst that could happen if he continued to process the target material. An intervention may go as follows:

CLIENT: Nothing is changing, I'm seeing Joe lying there with his head blown off.

THERAPIST: What do you imagine would be the worst thing that could happen if this material continued to process?

CLIENT: I might cry.

THERAPIST: What would be the problem with that?

CLIENT: I never let anybody see me cry. It's a sign of weakness.

THERAPIST: Where did you get that idea?

CLIENT: I don't remember. My father never cried, crying was just always not for men.

THERAPIST: What if I told you that crying is a normal release of emotion for men and women, and holding back sometimes can be bad for you? Holding back emotions can lead to a buildup that gets released in the kind of anger that you've talked about, that comes out when you don't expect it, and hurts people you don't want to hurt.

CLIENT: Yeah, intellectually I know that it's OK to cry, I just can't accept it.

THERAPIST: Would you be willing to put a picture in your mind of yourself crying and do eye movement?

There are a variety of different approaches that could have been taken here. Once the client said that crying was the issue, I chose to try to access early memories and beliefs, and then introduce what might be new information to begin to form a more positive associative network of different cognitions about crying. I could have, alternatively, asked the client to look for an incident, earlier in his life, around crying and made that a whole new target with the standard accessing methods. The result of any of these interventions might be rapid resolution of the initial problem, without the need for experiencing the sadness, or the result could be the client's experiencing the sadness and continuing to process.

The examples about crying and vulnerability touch on just one of many areas that may prevent processing with any client. Following are a number of specific associative networks in which combat veterans and others often get "stuck," sometimes not resolvable with changes in Category 3 activity. The elements described below are often closely interrelated, but even small differences can be important. For example, maintaining one's role as being damaged by the war may be important to one veteran because he cannot access any other more positive self-concept, but for another veteran the damaged role may be important because, if he does not see himself as damaged by events he participated in, he would powerfully access the idea that he is evil — because only an evil person could be undamaged by such events. While both cling to the role of damaged veteran, the information needed to resolve the problem is very different, as illustrated below.

While the following issues are usually not addressed until processing is blocked, it should also be noted that the material sometimes applies to the beginning of treatment, and therefore overlaps with the previous discussion of positive schema. Some of what is described below may prevent the client from initiating treatment and it may be helpful to allow the client to get started with other issues and come to these as they arise.

It should also be mentioned that these interventions are made in a conversational manner, as they would be in non-EMDR therapy, but with EM added at various times. They are also not made in isolation of each other, they are offered as hypotheses, and sometimes several are offered together if that seems clinically appropriate, then followed by Category 3 activity. The hope in giving several choices is that the client will be less likely to be blocked by his false belief[6] that the therapist is taking control.

By way of offering theoretical justification for multiple interpretations, I have recently come across reference to Kurt Lewin's concept of "channel factors" in behavior change (Ross and Nisbett, 1991) referring to details of a situation that, when addressed, can open up a path resulting in large changes. It may be that in offering a variety of hypotheses a channel will more likely be accessed, allowing for the large change that comes with integration. In retrospect the EMDR method of accessing a variety of associative network elements makes it more likely that a channel factor will be hit upon, resulting in rapid change not seen in methods limited to a narrower range.

On to the examples:

Need to maintain self-belief as war injured. A client may have little confidence that relief from PTSD symptoms will change his life circumstances. Even if he loses the nightmares or similar symptoms, he still has to live with the consequences of his reaction to the war, such as poor family, education, or vocational adjustment. Therefore, the symptoms may be frozen to maintain the status of being a "fucked-up combat vet." These symptoms carry inexplicable pain; however, this pain is preferable to the pain of being aware of the disarray of his life without intrusive symptoms as a reminder that it may not be his fault.

In a sense, the negative self-image of "fucked-up combat vet" has really served as a positive schema, substituting a "better" negative for a worse negative, such as being a failure or "scum." It is the tendency of combat veterans who have not psychologically recovered from war to be among the most profoundly self-denigrating people — part of what makes them so sensitive to criticism and rejection. Ascribing their problems to this "combat vet" identity is a move toward a more "positive" label, as well as a move in the direction of understanding their behavior as situationally determined, and therefore far superior to purely negative character explanations.

When a client reveals that leaving behind his combat veteran identity is an area of concern, one possible therapeutic approach is to try to access positive associative networks. Explore with the client any aspect of his current or recent life that was or is positive or that could become positive. When a client cannot or will not acknowledge any such possibility, I may ask for a recollection of some positive activity prior to the military. One client in an inpatient program, whom I was only briefly able to see, could acknowledge nothing positive in his life except bowling as a teenager. We made that the initial target of eye movement.

---

6. As most therapists know, and almost no clients deeply understand at the start of therapy, the therapist has almost no control of what is really important in therapy: the client making internal changes. The therapist has potential influence, but not control.

More typically and beneficially, I might help a client access memories of some period of positive functioning as an employee, parent, student, or spouse, and do EM with that memory. As we proceed, discussion might come to failures in the performance of that role; however, I would ask that we look carefully at these failures: almost always, they are attributable to some behavior that is modifiable and is often trauma related. This leaves open the possibility that trauma work will lead to not just losing the "fucked-up vet" role, but gaining a positive role. It may be important to also help introduce or access the role of well-functioning vet — one who retains his combat skills (including the skill to do nothing when action would be dangerous) for the rare but real possibility that they are needed. The issues presented in the next section, on connection to fellow veterans both living and dead, may become relevant here.

Another factor that helps to maintain the negative identity because positive self-schema are blocked from acceptance, is the memory of rejection or neglect when veterans came home, particularly, but not exclusively (see Severo and Milford 1989), from the Vietnam and Korean Wars. The most extreme examples are the incidents of Vietnam vets being spit upon or called "baby killers." Even veterans who were not so rejected received a powerful message when they were advised, after returning home, not to go out in their uniforms. Several African-American veterans have told me about being scorned in their own communities for fighting in the "white man's war." Veterans have also commonly told me how family appeared to reject them in other ways, telling them they were no longer the same person, with the clear statement or implication of being a worse person.[7] Employers, they often have said, would not hire them if they found out about their Vietnam service. The less virulent form of this phenomenon is apparent in frequent veteran complaints that, when they returned, no one wanted to talk with them about the war. Exposure to these kinds of events at times of extreme emotion could easily lead to building or reinforcing associative networks that include false information such as "Others reject me, so I am unacceptable, no good," and so forth.

For many veterans the resolution or correction of these networks includes the introduction of new information. Using Vietnam as an example, a therapist who is fully aware of the times can share the knowledge that the majority of people, and even the vast majority of war protesters, were certainly not against the servicemen. Explain how one or a few incidents of rejection could take on a dominant role for a person as vulnerable as a returning veteran, and *feel* as though it represented the truth. It may also be helpful to ask the veteran if he wanted to talk about the war, and explain the possible position of other people. I think it has been helpful for me to tell veterans how I, in my early twenties, seeing people I knew return from Vietnam, did not question them about it. I tell them how at the time I thought, and still think, that a person's activity in a war is one of the most

---

7. Likewise, veterans were often welcomed and/or had some people ready to listen, but the veteran was not ready to accept this response. When it is true, it is sometimes recognized in the course of therapy.

intimate and sensitive topics imaginable. And at that age I did not have the knowledge of life necessary to ask without being intrusive so, rather than risk causing pain, I remained silent unless the topic was brought up first by the veteran. As discussion of these matters occurs, the therapist should remain sensitive to points in which the processing of what is said or felt can be facilitated. The following interchange could occur after a brief discussion about how far back he could remember not having a way to talk and to be with people peacefully.

CLIENT: ...and nobody would talk to me about it. I just stayed in my room, ate, and went back to my room.

THERAPIST: Do you think they weren't interested, or do you think maybe they didn't know to ask or talk about something so painful?

CLIENT: I don't know.

THERAPIST: See what your brain does with it. (*Commence EM*)

CLIENT: Maybe they weren't rejecting me, they just couldn't cope with how I was then. (*Continuing EM*)

So ... I'm still stuck.

THERAPIST: If you were going to be with them differently, and talk to them, what is one positive way you could do that?

CLIENT: What do you mean? I don't know what you are talking about.

THERAPIST: Notice what you are feeling now. (*Continuing EM*)

CLIENT: I'm scared to talk to them, I don't know how. I've never really talked anywhere but here about the war.

From this point many directions are possible. With more EM the client may come up with a scenario, or realize that he still does not know what he wanted to say, or the therapist could do some assertive work with covert or actual role playing, and eye movement interspersed. If specific nonnegative identity behaviors can be practiced, pervasive elements such as general positive beliefs may be strengthened and make reprocessing of negative material more likely. Finally, this work might access specific war memories that require further processing by the veteran; he has to talk to himself about them before he can talk to anyone else.

*Pain and clear memories of combat are the client's only connection to his
friends.* He believes that if he loses the pain he loses, and perhaps even
dishonors, them. This is not an unusual dynamic for noncombat grief as
well. My clients often find it helpful in this situation to be asked to describe
a friend, his personality, what he liked about him. I ask how often these
positive qualities come up. Most clients say they are stuck in the memory
of the death. We may proceed thus:

THERAPIST: So when you think of Joe, do you think about him as the
person you liked and felt close to or about how he died?

CLIENT: How he died — that's about all I think of.

THERAPIST: How would you like to remember him? Would you prefer to
have your memory dominated by his life or by his death?

CLIENT: By his life.

THERAPIST: Start with that. (*Begin a set of EM*)

In helping clients with multiple losses of fellow adolescents, sometimes
in situations where the client believes he didn't do his best (to put it euphe-
mistically), I often rely on that timeless human concept, memorial. I ask
whether or not he believes he carries something of his friends with him.
Clients usually say they do and we discuss this.

THERAPIST: What do you think of the idea that your life is one of the ways
your friends still exist? In a sense it is a kind of memorial. Do you think
your friend(s) would want you to carry them around only experiencing
the pain? Would they want you to be self-destructive or to find some
positive sense of peace?[8]

CLIENT: I think they would want me to find some peace and happiness.

(*Depending on the flow of the conversation and nonverbal cues, I might then
ask the client to start with that and do EM, or I might say:*)

---

8. It may be that in this situation the client may take *peacefulness* to mean the peace that might
come with suicide and death; that is why I added the word *positive*. However, although clients
may have thought about "peace" self-destructively and discussed suicide with me at other
times, they have not in this context. Perhaps clients who have made it to this stage of therapy
have friends who wouldn't want this for them.
    I have had clients who, when we entered into a discussion like this, had "friends" who
would have promoted violence. As the discussion proceeds, they sometimes realize that they
weren't really that close to those friends. At other times I ask if they had lived, might not their
friend have grown to see life differently. I have also found it helpful to note that if violence
"worked" to resolve their distress, they wouldn't be coming for help — violence is what caused
their problems. The people for whom violence works well don't volunteer for therapy.

THERAPIST: Do you think a more positive life for yourself would be a better memorial for your friends than the way you have been living recently?

CLIENT: Yes.

THERAPIST: In your mind, would you talk to your friends about this and listen to what they might say, and then let's do some EM.

(Pause for a few seconds, then start to lead EM.)

Another belief that is part of this embittering negative network, and helps to maintain it, partly by the perpetuation of anger which interferes with accessing curative information, is that their friend died for nothing because the war was "lost" or because of the specific circumstances of their death. I don't agree with that position and I ask them why they and their friend went in the military. If the answer doesn't include some notion of duty or responsibility, I ask about it specifically. I might ask:

THERAPIST: Did your friend go in to do right or wrong?

CLIENT: Right.

THERAPIST: How would he have felt about himself if he went to Canada?

CLIENT: He couldn't have done it.

THERAPIST: So one of the true ways to look at this is that your friend died because he went in the military, and he did that because it was right. So no matter how your friend died in the war, he died because he did the right thing, and to not be there would have been wrong for him. He did not die for nothing. Notice what happens. (*Commence EM*)

If my client can see that his friend did not die for nothing, some of the pain will be resolved.

In addressing this issue I have also raised the question how and when one decides what the meaning of an event is. The idea of our making of meaning was discussed in a previous section around dealing with the meaning of the Vietnam War, and death in it. Just as the meaning of the war changes over time, so do the meanings of all kinds of events. The therapist can choose one event from the client's life or history to illustrate.[9]

9. Some teachers of psychotherapy might say that this type of political discussion has no place in treatment. I disagree; the best advice I received when I started working with combat veterans was that I would have to break down some of the normal barriers between client and therapist if we were to get any work done at all.

Pain and suffering of the symptoms of PTSD are the client's connection to his own humanity. This applies most strongly when the client has behaved in a regrettable way, which in war can mean anything. In such a circumstance comfort, especially acknowledging any comfort, leads to associations of even more extreme negative self-evaluation. In this regard, I sometimes ask clients to consider ideas discussed in Chapter 4 in the section about positive schema and spirituality. Ideas about human nature, discussion of psychology research by Milgram (1974) on how easily people adapt to situational norms and authority, even when destructive violation of basic beliefs are involved, are also sometimes helpful to clients. The idea of growth and human potential can also be helpful.

Another frequently useful approach is to go back to the events leading up to the target behavior. Almost invariably, clients who have profound guilt about their actions that did not come from following orders experienced great loss or terror prior to their regretted action: a close friend was killed or maimed, or they witnessed American victims of atrocities. When working with a client on his own regretted behavior who is stuck, I probe for his loss and try to target that with EM. This will sometimes provide some relief on the original target.

Another way in which events in war may unfold to lead clients to horrible treatment of others is when a soldier decided during the war that he was *certainly* not going to survive, and took his revenge before the fact. My guess is that most people who reached that conclusion probably did die because of enemy action, or arranged to die to keep their part of the bargain made in their own mind. Some were wounded or for other reasons escaped a certain death, and are being treated for PTSD. This is a dynamic that I believe I have witnessed but not yet had the opportunity to address overtly with Category 3 activity.

Ego-syntonic aspects of war. In addition to symptoms, the war provided some people with their first and sometimes only chance to feel powerful. In many cultures, including many parts of ours, small boys learn that the only true path to power and respect is that of being a warrior, or athlete, or tough guy, or gangster. I had a client who stopped moving his eyes and began to act as if he were engaged in driving a tank. I vigorously attempted to get him to begin moving his eyes again and to break through and reorient him. He interrupted his "driving" to tell me to leave him alone. This type of event has been extremely rare during the EM process, but others have talked about the issue of how inadequate or cowardly they felt before the service and how they don't intend to be in those roles again.

The weaker and more common form of this dynamic often occurs after some processing when the client is at a decreased, but still high, level of discomfort. Clients sometimes say that if they continue the work and become calm, they will lose the "edge" that protected them during and since the war. When this issue arises, I initiate a discussion about arousal levels and which are most protective. I might even cite the Yerkes-Dodson Law, which includes the idea that sometimes lower levels of arousal promote better performance than higher levels of arousal (Wolman, 1977), thereby giving the weight of authority to my opinion.

Through conversation and questioning, we usually determine that the client's current level of arousal has led to more dangerous situations, and has not been as protective as a lower level would be. It is acknowledged, however, that in combat, on guard duty, or when "walking point," a much higher level of arousal is required than that safest for walking in the shopping mall. (When talking about tension reduction, I do not make "relaxation" the goal.) I then ask the client what level of tension he considers optimal; specifically, I might ask: "Could you feel safe at a lower level than where you are now?" If the client says "yes," I might just say: "Start with that" and begin a set of eye movements, and continue with processing and accessing.

The therapist must be aware that, in addition to the stated need for arousal, a feeling of comfort or being relaxed may be aversive. This is even true in the general population. Several studies have reported clients showing increased distress with traditional relaxation exercises (Heide and Borkovec, 1984; see Lichstein, 1988, for a review). A client may have had disastrous events occur in combat or have heard of such things occurring to soldiers who were relaxed. These situations, if they can be identified, may be good processing targets to further access.

Continued processing of a target trauma may lead to other remembered or "sensed" painful events. This is among the most difficult types of progress blocks to deal with. One way to discover this is to ask specifically if it is the case. If the client indicates it is, the Category 3 activity should stop and the possible consequences of proceeding should be discussed again. In my experience and that of my colleagues, when this occurs the material blocked from processing most often, but not always, has a perpetrator or felt perpetrator aspect to it. I might say to a client:

THERAPIST: Sometimes when clients get to this point, the things they don't want to explore involve something they did or think they did to others. It often involves guilt and shame. I'm not asking you to reveal any events now, but what do you think of what I just said?

CLIENT: It might have something to do with that.

THERAPIST: What are the potential life paths for someone who has done, or been part of, something horrible?

(This is the time to access the points discussed in previous sections about positive schema and forgiveness.)

The pain associated with trauma has served as justification for subsequent otherwise unacceptable behavior, so the relief of this discomfort would increase guilt feelings. I sometimes see the dynamic (associative pattern) in which the client has been a substance abuser and an irresponsible or cruel parent or spouse. Over the course of treatment, the client may develop the intellectual insight that this behavior is connected to the reaction to war. For these clients, resolution of war-related problems, especially intrusive memories, may leave them feeling increased guilt. When this is the situation, it may be helpful to target more recent material related to post-war adjustment or, rather, failure to adjust.

The issues of government and country constitute mixed schema for many combat veterans; giving up anger, as occurs with processing of trauma, in addition to making the client more vulnerable to painful emotions, may place him in the position of forgiving when he doesn't want to. Clients for whom processing is blocked, who have expressed strong anger at the government in general conversation, may need to deal with this issue to progress, even if it does not come up at the time processing is blocked.

In this context it is sometimes important to remind the client that forgiveness does not mean everything is right, it may only mean that other areas of the relationship can take center stage again.

I think it may also be helpful for clients to consider the nature of the relationship between the nation, its leadership, and its people in general. I ask the client to consider the proposition that we form our relationship with the nation and government as children, and the government then is seen as a parent, a protector who can also punish. Even if the government is seen in a negative light (for example, the police are seen as "The Man" rather than "Officer Friendly"), it is still a parental light and we hope that we can have this bad parent become a good one. When our view of the relationship with this parent is one of betrayal, we may become enraged — to give up this rage takes away our only means of protest to the powerful bad parent. Emotional conflict comes into play because, even with the most severely abusive parent, there is attachment and loyalty by the child. So it is with the government that is seen as a betrayer, as is particularly the case among Vietnam and Korean War veterans.

If the client is still with me, I go on to describe how — in the normal course of events as we mature — it is best to begin to see the government as our child, rather than as our parent. Outside the war context, this transition is accomplished gradually: we see the government as our creation as we pay taxes, vote, serve on PTAs, or involve ourselves in political activities. As with the actual children we raise, we have influence but we can't maintain complete control. Perhaps most important from a psychological point of view, we hope the country/government will, like a child, carry on the best we are after we are gone. Finally, I might explain how it is natural and adaptive for the parent to ultimately love the child more than the child loves the parent. After all, in the usual scheme of things the parent forms his attachment when the child is young, and the parent does not have to limit attachment to prepare fully for the loss of the child in the same way as the child lives his life preparing for independence and the loss of the parent. When seen this way, the nation and its leadership can still legitimately hold our attachment, even when — like an errant child — it "betrays" us. In this context, we can perhaps forgive it for what we hope it will become.

When a person sees the worst of the government in its bad parent role, such as was seen during the Vietnam War in particular, it is very difficult to make the relationship transition. The betrayed party is stuck in the child position and in rage. I ask clients to consider the perspective, discuss it, and then do Category 3 activity.

Clients are stuck on a negative self-belief that they can intellectually see is untrue from some perspectives, but remains true from others. The acceptance of the changed perspective cannot be accomplished because it would subvert a highly valued world view. The negative cognition of "coward" often sticks with an incident in which the client momentarily "froze," even when he intellectually understands the biological determinants of the momentary inaction. I try to help clients see that the all-or-none labeling and extreme name calling in the military — as well as by parents and other authorities — is motivational speech, and is often not even intended to be accurate, or generalized to other situations. This extreme judgmental way of looking at people and the world is for crises, or to prevent crises, not to live by in day-to-day civilian life; it is essentially useless for post-situation analysis. After the crisis is over, good military men don't spend much time sitting around labeling — they try to figure out how to do it better next time. They determine what aspects of training were helpful, what need to be changed, and how. When it appears a client is stuck in this manner, we discuss these ideas and then proceed with Category 3 behavior. Category 3 behavior, as with other discussion-type interweaves, is requested whether or not the client agrees with the analysis. The client is asked to begin with the idea and see what happens next.

I see this variation of cognitive therapy as a Category 2 activity that respects the military (or parenting/schooling) experience, yet allows the client to integrate a more adaptive element in the target network.

As can be seen in the list of network elements that might impede processing of trauma, it would be almost impossible, early in the treatment process, to meet the goal of identifying the most salient negative and positive cognitions for the complex and distant trauma that one might find in treating war veterans and other trauma victims. It is often only after processing begins that the salient negative elements are accessed and "solution" elements can be accessed or introduced. However, in beginning the intensive trauma phase of treatment, where Category 3 activity will be initiated, it is wise to start with standard EMDR accessing protocols to maximize the efficiency of treatment.

chapter 6

End of Session, End of Treatment

Ending a Session

The discussion in Chapter 5 centered on how to foster therapeutic processing and overcome blocked processing. The next question concerns how it is decided that work on a traumatic event is complete and, if it is not, how to end the session.

Shapiro (1995) delineates clear criteria to judge complete processing of a specific event. When the work on a traumatic event or other target, such as a specific fear, results in the client coming to a relaxed state when fully contemplating it, when associated stimuli do not produce maladaptive reactions, and when the client fully accepts neutral or positive ideas about himself in the context of the event, processing is complete. While this kind of resolution is common for many clients in other settings, it is rare to fully process a traumatic event in a single session — or even a few sessions — for clients with chronic combat-related PTSD who come to the DVA for outpatient treatment.

I have come to expect that processing will not be complete enough in an individual session for me to use the first standard test of having the client go back to the original target. Most sessions end with the client far more comfortable than at the beginning of the session, but still with more processing to do on the target. For the majority of clients, I do not use formal calming exercises to end the session. The natural course seems to be for clients to end the session with more comfort, new insight, and sustained involvement in continuing processing on their own before the next session. I don't view each therapy session as a discrete episode, but rather as part of a continuing effort by the client to integrate his experience, as well as part of a sustained conversation between us. If there is a Category 4 activity at the end of most sessions, it is conversation about the client's plans for the day or some other subject of mutual interest removed from the work of the session.

Incomplete Processing

There are several possible reasons, aside from the complexity of each traumatic event (addressed in previous sections), why some clients do not complete processing an event in one — or even two or three — sessions:

1. War-related trauma is often not organized discretely; one event leads into another. I usually follow the client's flow of these events because most clients find a natural pause where discomfort abates and trauma work can be interrupted. Even though the second time a series of events is targeted the absolute level of distress may be lower all along the stream of images, it is still important to end at a level relatively low for that session. There are a few clients, however, for whom there are so many events connected together, with no decrease in distress, that I will ask the client to consider allowing us to focus on one event and bring him back to it when he moves away from it.

2. Most sessions are an hour or less, as opposed to the 90 minutes recommended by Shapiro. My initial sessions that include Category 3 activity are almost always scheduled for at least 90 minutes. I continue to schedule sessions of 90 minutes or more for clients who cannot reach comfortable stopping points in less time, but work on trauma is always discussed and scheduled in the previous session with these clients. For the majority of clients who are able to work in blocks of time of an hour or less, trauma work is usually not scheduled. The client decides in each session what would be most useful for him. Which brings us to the next point.

3. For the vast majority of my clients the trauma and symptoms directly related to it, such as nightmares and intrusive thoughts, are just one part of the problem. These veterans might have been able to simply focus on trauma work if they had been effectively treated soon after the war (had an effective treatment been available); however, the intervening years have led to a multitude of problems, often the result of efforts to decrease the effects of the initial response to trauma. Counseling sessions must address substance abuse, anger management, family, employment, and other social issues, or the alliance will be broken because the client will, correctly, believe that I am not recognizing the hierarchy of his needs. These other issues can often be addressed with Category 3 activity, but usually must wait for, or be interspersed with, extensive work in the other categories; for example, the Category 2 activity of teaching assertiveness (see Appendix 1, Feelings Identification and Behavioral Rehearsal). To be more explicit, a client may work on a trauma during one session, in the next session talk about the work's effect on him, and then focus on a family or job issue. Eye movement or other Category 3 activity may be used with a target from the family or job issue, or other more conventional therapeutic activity may take place.

4. Outpatient work in a DVA medical center may have both advantages and disadvantages compared to the private sector or to other not-for-profit settings. The client's identification of the treatment facilitator with the perpetration of the original trauma and competing motivational issues have been discussed. On the other hand, as of this writing most of my clients do not have to have approval from an administrator for more than a handful of counseling sessions. The right to treatment, especially for clients whose problems are recognized by the DVA as resulting from military service, is established. Therefore, there is no bureaucratic or personal financial reason why most clients must limit therapy. Their problems are therefore not defined narrowly and counseling can be comprehensive enough to thoroughly work through problems, or even to provide extended consultative services.

Amount and Type of Trauma

Absent from this list of factors that leads to less likelihood of single-session processing for combat veterans than for most other clients is premorbid adjustment. There have been many studies examining why one combat veteran has more postcombat psychological problems than another (Goldberg et al. 1990; King et al. 1996; Lee et al. 1995).

While there is some divergence of opinion, the most powerful case can be made for the position that amount and type of trauma are the most important determinants. If precombat psychological problems do explain much of the differences, we don't know which factors these are. This also reflects my clinical impression. Overall, my clients with severe combat PTSD symptoms appear to have premilitary adjustment comparable to clients with less severe problems. In general, my clients, both those who are severely and less severely impacted, appear to have premilitary adjustment similar to the population as a whole. I believe the main difference in the effect of combat trauma, aside from amount of trauma, is the *specific meaning of the trauma* to the client. That is, the nature of the networks formed to account for the events and the meaning of the events themselves. For example, one episode of teenage socially pressured, personal-loss-precipitated cruelty may be enough to cause severe symptoms in a premorbidly highly moral, conventionally well-adjusted veteran who views his transgression as an inexcusable violation of his values, whereas a similar event may have less effect on a veteran with a less prosocially structured belief system.

Termination of Therapy

The successful completion of psychotherapy is most fruitfully talked about in terms of the meeting of goals. Earlier, the goals of psychotherapy were defined in general, from the point of view of the FAM, to be the completion of information processing. The exception to this is the intermediate goal of limiting the accessing of information (that is, anxiety, rage, or other emotions that may be immediately destructive). This abstract expression of goals may shed light on the overall therapy process, but does not do much to clarify the nature of any one client/therapist contract. It is the fulfillment of that contract or, alternatively, the overt decision to abandon it, that leads to the formal termination of therapy.

There are several different goals that can be established between the client and therapist, ranging from long-term supportive counseling to short-term symptom reduction. In establishing goals, various combinations of processing and limiting of accessing are used.

For the clients described previously who participated in EMDR and Category 3 activity, one goal was clearly the processing of information — or, in client terms, relief of troublesome problem(s) such as excessive rage or nightmares, through work on the underlying events that caused these problems. When the client reports that these goals are met and the therapist's observation concurs, the discussion of other goals takes place. This work includes the recognition of previously only implicitly stated goals, such as those relating to family or employment problems; work now begins with this new set of goals or termination begins.

Evaluating Goal Attainment

As all therapists know, clients must be asked to explore resolution of symptoms in detail because superficial relief may mask work that still needs to be done. At the same time, the inexperienced EMDR therapist especially must be careful not to assume that quick results are superficial. As in most things, too much emphasis on one or the other extreme is not good.

When checking the result of the therapeutic work, it is essential to follow Shapiro's recommendation of asking the client to go through the target events in as much detail as possible and to observe for distress, as well as for likely future trigger situations. An additional effective way to test for thoroughness of completion is to engage the client in discussion of aspects of the target problem that have not been worked with at all. If the client cannot consider the target events for discussion in the same way he would consider other non-symptom-producing events, the work is not complete. (Of course, if the client decides the therapy is terminated, then therapy is terminated with the work incomplete.)

The following is an example of more fully evaluating the therapy work for a client who has completely processed the death of a friend in a battle. If he can imagine the battle from start to finish and remain peaceful (not numb), I may then ask him to talk about his friend:

THERAPIST: Tell me about Joe. What was he like as a person?

CLIENT: You know, in some ways we didn't know each other very well, but I remember he liked music.

THERAPIST: What kind of music?

CLIENT: You know, rock-and-roll.

THERAPIST: What are some of the songs that you remember hearing or talking about with him?

CLIENT: A lot of Motown, the Temptations, things like that.

THERAPIST: Have you ever run across anyone who looked like him?[1]

CLIENT: I don't know, let me think … the last time I saw him, he didn't look like anybody at all…

THERAPIST: Right now, on that 0 to 10, where are you?

CLIENT: A lot of the anxiety is back, 6.

At this point there should be sufficient rapport to simply ask the client to note his experience and begin EM again. That is done and the associations are followed until completion, when standard procedures and discussion are again initiated to evaluate processing.

The decision that processing of an event is complete cannot rest on the idea that there will never be any emotion in response to war-related material. It is expected that clients will retain appropriate emotion; viewing a film about the war can be expected to produce a stronger reaction than it might in the population at large, but it should not be of debilitating magnitude. It is difficult to be clear about the difference between a normal emotional response and a maladaptive one. Some questions that may help to differentiate are:

Does the client experience it as an emotion or a symptom?
Does it interfere with normal functioning?
Does it persist?
Does it lead to negative self-beliefs?
Is it experienced as a reaction to a memory or as part of reexperiencing?
Can it produce insight or understanding?

When the client is no longer distressed by stimuli related to the target, it is still wise to ask him to be particularly aware of anniversary times or holidays for increased distress. It is sometimes the case that particular dates or times of year will trigger responses that could not be accessed for treatment during the course of therapy. (The importance of reminding clients to prepare for anniversary dates was emphasized for me by Dan Merlis and

---

1. When there is good rapport, this kind of sudden change in direction is common and is usually more fluid and acceptable in conversation than it reads.

Gene Schwartz.) There may be other unanticipated stimuli that cause problems for a client and it is important that he understand that the retriggering of the problem is not failure of the therapy but, rather, the feedback that it was not complete. The more the client understands intellectually about the way the mind works in acquiring problems and relieving them, the easier this work is to do and to complete.

In the VA system where I have done the vast majority of my clinical work, clients may expect that therapy is not time limited or tied to the processing of only one problem. This is especially true for clients who are officially rated "disabled,"[2] whether or not they are vocationally and socially functioning at very high levels. For clients officially rated disabled, there is the institutionalized expectation that the disability may lessen in severity but will not disappear, that it is "permanent." Given the state of knowledge about the treatment of PTSD up until the last few years, the expectation of symptom permanence was reasonable. It is still reasonable to believe that, even if they are helped substantially — I have seen retired World War II and Korean War veterans benefit from EMDR — no psychotherapy will make the majority of middle-aged or older, severe chronic combat PTSD clients vocationally and socially uninjured after many years of being affected by symptoms.

Clients whose initial goal in treatment is to process trauma may also have established the goal of processing current events as they arise. Other clients, described previously in the discussion of ways in which to encourage acceptance of EMDR, have more limited goals: they may likewise want to diminish the effects of past trauma; however, they are also concerned that in the course of this work their level of distress never rise above some feared point.[3] Another way of saying this is that they must always perceive themselves as in control, a reasonable requirement for people who associate being out of control with killing or other dangerous actions. The effect of this goal is that processing must go forward with only limited accessing of traumatic events or using Category 3 activity, as these increase the risk of distress and feared loss of control.

Counter-Transference Concerns

Again, as all therapists know, the therapist's goals can at times interfere with therapy. Termination is one area in which my underlying beliefs are more likely to influence my position than in other areas.

I would agree with a client's plan to extend therapy beyond the achievement of the goal of complete processing of trauma, even if I were not part

2. Disability ratings in the DVA system for problems that have roots in military service are determined by percent of impairment. The guidelines are too involved to explain here; however, a veteran who has some symptoms of a problem such as PTSD, but who is functioning well in many dimensions, may be considered "disabled," but at a 0% or 10% level. This may help to guarantee the veteran treatment for the aspects of the problem that may emerge.
3. This is a reasonable concern for veterans who have acted violently in response to trauma-related stimuli.

of an organization that I believe has responsibility to clients beyond resolving specific symptoms. This belief that the organization that employs me has an obligation beyond that of the conventional private practice obligation is one point that causes me to watch for countertransference issues in goal setting. The other is that, despite my strong professional belief and stated position that the client defines the work, I am very ambitious for my clients and, in my heart of hearts, I want them all to attain a level of integration, serenity, and self-actualization that may not exist, although I certainly hope it does.[4] By this standard, our work is never complete: we can always target a new potential source of discomfort and better integrate a positive schema that will ward off *any* anxiety. In conflict with this wish for my clients is my observation of myself and others, even acknowledged master psychotherapists and profoundly advanced spiritualists, that is in line with that of May and Yalom (1995): "...anxiety is a part of existence and no individual who continues to grow and create will ever be free of it." (p. 286) So the client who has met our stated goal, but who still has some anxiety, may be making the most appropriate decision when he terminates therapy.

Thus, when my client and I end regular appointments either by mutual agreement or with the client telling me he does not wish another appointment, I hope my client will not run into difficulties that he is not prepared to cope with. I always tell the client that, if he wishes to make use of my knowledge in the future, I will try to be available. I try to get across the message that the use of my services does not imply illness or weakness; in fact, the desire to use my services in the future may be a sign of strength.

This position is consistent with a point I make to help some clients be more accepting of therapy at the beginning of treatment: that all people have the innate need to share their experience with others who understand — in a sense, people from their "neighborhood," people with whom they share a lot of assumptions. When someone has been to war, it is difficult to find people from that "neighborhood" in day-to-day life and, even when he does, he knows that sharing may often be intrusion. Therefore, people who have been through such experiences may need to see someone like myself to meet this basic human need, someone who — even if he has not been there — knows enough about the "neighborhood" to be able to listen intelligently.

---

4. I know I haven't achieved it either, although, for at least two reasons, it would be better if I did. First, the obvious selfish reason. Second, after being closely involved in the training of hundreds of therapists as they learn to apply EMDR with each other, it seems that we *tend* to not expect or work toward clients being psychologically "better" than we are. I have seen many EMDR therapists-in-training begin to stop the therapy process when the practicum "client" reached a level of anxiety with the target material that the therapist believed was the best one could expect. Very often, just the brief supervisory suggestion that EM continue resulted in lower anxiety and even a positive reconsideration of the target event. So, the "better" I am, the less likely it is that I will unintentionally limit my clients' evolution to the level that I would be happy with for myself.

Outcome

This book, as well as most psychotherapy texts, contains case studies to illustrate one point or another, or controlled research studies testing a therapeutic approach in a setting not dissimilar to a genuine clinical setting that is also tainted by a "research" rather than a therapeutic relationship. Therefore, one never gets a truly objective reading of the author's therapeutic results in his or her general practice.

I was hoping to do evaluation differently in this book. To that end, I initiated a survey in April 1997 of 30 clients with whom I had at least one individual therapy session in the month of February 1995. The results were generally positive but, because of the low (nine clients) response rate, the results are of very limited scientific use. I have decided not to report specifics because to do so might give the appearance that I thought I — unlike colleagues criticized earlier for their reports — had made an objective evaluation on my clinical practice. Consequently, I will simply climb into the basket of psychotherapist writers and claim that my clients benefit significantly from my work, without offering objective evidence, only a general overall impression.

The results of my clinical work do appear both generally positive to me and to have improved over time, as I learned and offered clients what I have presented in the preceding chapters. Some clients report and demonstrate such positive gains as losing "startle responses" or reactivity to formerly provocative stimuli such as helicopters. I have had clients return to employment and sustain abstinence from drugs and/or alcohol for "record" lengths of time. On the other hand, a few clients who have begun treatment that included Category 3 have symptoms that appeared to be impervious to my best efforts; a few improved, but refused to continue beyond one session with Category 3 activity. A small number of clients have begun treatment, accessed more trauma than they had in the past, then refused to continue Category 3 activity, which left some of them with more intrusive symptoms than in the past. Most of these clients continue to pursue treatment that does not include overt Category 3 activity. What I want to convey here is that the suggestions I have offered in the previous chapters have mostly "worked" but sometimes they haven't, and sometimes when they have I didn't know which ones did the job.

Leaving on this note of uncertainty seems fitting to me. If the best of psychotherapy is, as I claim earlier, about enhancing information processing for our clients, then it is not about making them well, but rather it is about helping them be better prepared for the uncertainty of the futures we all face.

Appendix 1

Feelings Identification and Behavioral Rehearsal (FIBRe) Group

This appendix is the client manual for an instruction/role-play group that I have been offering to clients for several years. It is based on the well-known concept that, the vast majority of the time, when anger or emotional numbness occur — feelings that have often been destructive to my clients in peacetime adjustment — there is another, more primary, emotion such as fear, grief, or guilt that underlies the anger or numbness. I present the standard therapeutic ideas that it is in the client's best interest to identify this underlying emotion and find a way, when it is safe to do so, to name it, either directly to the person to whom it relates, to a supportive person, or at least to a diary.

I recognize that, for some clients, anger exists but is not acknowledged or displayed, and may be viewed by the therapist as a primary underlying emotion to depression. However, colleagues who often work with clients who have survived chronic abuse, who do not show anger, also report that it is common to find another "layer" of emotion, such as grief, beyond the anger, and that it is accessed in the completion of processing.

This material is included as one potentially useful non-EMDR-format example of the introduction of new information and/or making already known information more accessible for processing. It can be adapted to use in individual trauma-processing sessions. FIBRe may also serve as a Category 4 activity to simply reduce distress in difficult situations.

FIBRE Group Feelings Identification and Behavioral Rehearsal
— Howard Lipke, Ph.D.

In our relationships with others, there are times when we have strong reactions; at these times, our behavior can take one of three basic forms:

1. *Aggressive*: attacking another person to defeat them. This is sometimes the best thing to do in combat situations. Problems arise, however, when we attack in noncombat situations, often turning them into combat situations.

2. *Avoidant*: withdrawal, either physical or psychological. This is sometimes the best thing to do in combat situations, or to avoid turning a situation into a combat situation. Avoidance activities can range from emotional numbing and retreat from other people to meditation and relaxation exercises.

3. *Assertive*: expressing one's own position. The goal is not to defeat[1] another person, but rather to make sure that one's own point of view is expressed. There are basically three types of assertiveness:

> *Gathering information*: further exploring the situation to check on your
> initial impression of what occurred.
> *Assertion of rights and opinions*: telling others what you think.
> *Assertion of emotions*: telling others what you feel, which is far more
> difficult than the assertion of rights. Assertion of emotion is what
> FIBRe is about.

FIBRe group focuses on assertion of emotions, and has many parts, of which these three are essential:

1. The identification of emotions
2. The statement of emotions, especially those leading up to anger
3. The practice of the first two parts

Perhaps the best way to further explain this group is in the form of a dialogue, as follows.

> *Why should we bother to engage in these activities?*
>
> Very often, veterans who come for counseling do not participate in an activity that is conducive to improved physical health, peace of mind, and better social relations. That activity is the *statement of emotions*. And, logically, if emotions are to be stated they must first be *identified*. The practice element is important because, when learning and using any skill, whether it is firing a weapon, driving a car, or expressing yourself, *practice with feedback is essential for mastery.*
>
> *Why aren't emotions identified?*
>
> There are several reasons for this. First, in order to be identified an emotion must be experienced, rather than blocked or "numbed

---

1. Some people might criticize this as a "loser's" approach, but my observation is that it is more likely that goals will be accomplished if you focus on doing the best you can, not on defeating someone else.

out." For many combat veterans, emotions other than anger are often extremely painful and therefore blocked out. Sadness is often connected to the overpowering events of traumatic loss. Puzzlement, uncertainty, disappointment, worry, fear, and frustration are associated with the appearance of weakness, and could lead to danger in a combat situation. More pleasant emotions are also avoided because, in combat situations, one learns that feeling good, getting close to people by sharing happiness or fondness, leaves you open to greater pain when loss occurs. (Ironically, some people accept the good emotions that accompany substance abuse, because when these occur in the presence of alcohol or drugs, very little attachment is made to another person so there is less sense of vulnerability.) While many people with PTSD report that they do not have emotions other than rage, my experience with combat veterans, as well as research on physiological responses, shows the emotions are still there, but they are hidden.

Even though anger may be a serious problem, it may be useful to consider *anger and rage as a solution, rather than a problem*. Thus, if anger and rage are to be present less often, a person must be prepared for emotions such as sadness or worry. The benefit of being aware of these emotions is that one can make peace with things that cause them, or at least not be ambushed by the anger that comes up to block them. It should also be mentioned that many people, when they think of emotion, think of "fight or flight." They therefore think that "flight" is the same as fear and "fight" is the same as anger. In fact, fight and flight are *both reactions to fear*, which may next be experienced as anger and fight, or stay fear and result in flight.

How is FIBRe any different from other assertiveness training?

FIBRe is different from most assertiveness groups in that, usually, those groups concentrate on asserting rights or opinions, while FIBRe focuses on asserting emotions. Although the behaviors practiced in this group may help someone get what they want from others, that is a secondary goal. The reasons for the focus on emotions are:

1. The failure to assert emotions appropriately when they come up leads to "blowups" that are extremely destructive to meeting important life goals.
2. Failure to state emotions can lead to physical illness.
3. Statement of emotion helps clarify thoughts and situations.
4. Success in statement of emotions doesn't depend very much on others' cooperation.

This group does include some focus on getting others to act in one way or another; however, again, this is secondary in FIBRe, and should be worked on in other therapy situations. Another way to look at FIBRe is in terms of Reinhold Niebuhr's Serenity Prayer "...grant me the serenity to accept the things I cannot change, courage to change the things that I can, and wisdom to know the difference..." FIBRe is one way of working toward the first part, accepting the things that cannot be changed.

Why practice?

FIBRe emphasizes practice because the identification and statement of emotions is considered a skill. Just as with any other skill, such as driving a car or firing a weapon, practice is essential. Practice using the "not real" situation of role play is especially important, because this is a skill that needs to be used under stressful conditions. So, like initial driving lessons or weapons training, the skill must first be practiced in a somewhat controlled setting. You don't practice in "live" conditions.

When somebody is really giving me a hard time, this won't help, will it?

One frequent objection to the teaching of this skill is that it doesn't do any good on the "street." If what is meant by "street" is combat-like conditions, that is true. The VA does not offer combat training; our veterans are already certainly better at this than the nonveteran staff. However, long experience has taught counselors that most interpersonal problem situations do not occur in street confrontations, but rather with people such as family, friends, employers, and employees (including doctors, nurses, and clerical staff, among others).

So, what do you actually do in this group?

In this group we will be working from a formula that helps learning, and promotes using the skill. *First*, it is extremely important to *politely ask the listener* if he or she is available to converse. Then this formula asks group members to respond to the practice situation by *honestly speaking emotions* (and thoughts) *about a behavior or situation so that others can or will want to hear*, and (when necessary) *request behavior change. Listen for the response.*

Politely Ask for Listener Attention

This is the step that causes the most controversy. Some people think this is unnecessary and makes you look weak. I suggest it be done for at least three reasons:

1. If someone had something important to tell you, you would probably want them to politely get your attention. This step models for them the respect you want shown to you.

2. If they can't listen to you at the moment because they are distracted by the need to attend to something else, it gives you a chance to reschedule the conversation or choose a different way to deal with the situation.

3. Most people function in semitrances. We often don't hear things we don't expect to hear. You can probably think of times where someone said something to you and you didn't notice; that is true of others also. So if you ask someone if they are ready to listen and wait for the response, their response helps break the trance. (You may have noticed that some of the time when you have gotten what you wanted by acting angry, it wasn't always because of the other person's fear; sometimes it was because it broke the trance they were in.)

Honestly Speak Emotions

Honestly: If it is not honest, then it is impossible to accomplish the goal of statement of feelings. Although your statement must be honest, that doesn't mean that everything you believe must be stated. This is especially true of anger. Experience has made it clear that anger or rage usually are secondary emotions that follow quickly after fear or disappointment. It is important to identify these other related emotions and to express them when they are primary.

Speak: People often figure that others can guess how they feel, and therefore they shouldn't have to state the emotions. However, for many reasons, our emotions are not clear to others. People are blessed with language. A basic idea of this group is to help people use that ability in a constructive way.

Emotions (and thoughts): For all the reasons mentioned above, as well as for at least one more. When we state our emotions, we draw attention to the bond of humanity we share with others. We may have different thoughts, abilities, or appearances from others, but emotion is something we all share. When we talk of our own emotions, others can hear us better.

Focus, Request, Response

About a behavior or situation: If we focus on the other person, our communication will likely be heard as a judgment, and cause the person to either stop listening or start trying to protect herself or himself. In addition, we will often be wrong. It is impossible to sum up people, with all our complexities, with simple labels.

So that others can or want to hear: This refers to many factors, such as word order, posture, and nearness. Putting yourself in someone else's face will make the most pleasant words difficult to hear, as will a harsh tone of voice. Included in this section is the idea that the communication should be relatively brief, with the emotion expressed early and clearly.

Request behavior change (when necessary): If it is necessary to request behavior change, the principles stated above should be used.

Listen for the response: This may be the hardest part of all. When people are feeling strong emotions, even after they have stated them, those emotions tend to block out everything else. Listening for the response gives new information a chance to come in and enables emotions to change, sometimes even for the better.

What do you do when it doesn't work?

There are circumstances in which this or any effort might not work, and your response will depend on which way assertiveness didn't work. One kind of response to have in your repertoire is to repeat the process, focusing on the new emotion that comes up when your first statement of emotion didn't "work." Remember, even if the other person does not respond in the way you wish, at least you expressed your emotion. Remember, also, that unless you listen carefully to both the other person and your own emotions you won't know if it "worked."

Another way in which it might not work is if that person is not prepared to listen. In that case you may be better off using a calming exercise (avoidance of reaction) and then later find someone who can listen to you talk about your emotion. FIBRe can often help outside the situation in which the emotions occurred.

Won't saying how I feel leave me vulnerable?

In some ways, and in some situations, possibly. However, the need to hide feelings usually leaves you far more vulnerable. When people have something to hide they are always running scared, or angry, that someone may find out. If you say your feelings, you don't have to go through all kinds of maneuvers to hide them. In addition, most of the time other people can figure out that you have emotions, so the only one you are really fooling is yourself.

The plan of this group is to use the material to practice on realistic situations, with the goal of having these skills available to use if you so desire. Various situations will be discussed in group, with some opportunities to practice. You will then be given the chance for individual practice with staff during the week, so that different types of situations (and different types of responses from the other person) can be mastered.

There are many situations in which FIBRe can't be used because they are potential combat situations, or because you are just not ready at that time. Once you are out of the situation it can be helpful to identify and share your feelings with someone you do trust. Although this may not be as effective as saying it in the situation, it can work.

I know this guy who tried FIBRe once. He did everything you said, and the other person just got pissed off and left.

I know that guy, too, and what happened was that, later on, the other person told him that he was acting so different she just didn't believe him. That happens sometimes, and occasionally the other person is right — the person using FIBRe is just using it to run a game. If you practice enough, are honest, and stick with it, I think most people will respond positively. You won't know for sure unless you try.

Is there anything you would like to add about secondary goals or other motives?

Yes, but first I need to tell a story. Minnie told Joe she would be home at 10. At 11, she comes in looking tired. He says, "It really worries me when you tell me you're going to be home at 10, and look here," he points at his watch, "it's 11, and you're just now walking in the door." Minnie responds, "You asshole, you are always late."

Human communication is rarely simple, and we all act based on more than one motivation or goal. Even if statement of emotion is the *primary goal*, there may still be additional, sometimes hidden, goals within that — or any — communication. In the story of Minnie and Joe, Joe could claim that his primary goal was to tell Minnie he was worried. Even if we accept this as true, it looks like Joe is making other communications which, in FIBRe, are called *secondary goals*.

Some secondary goals support the primary goal and others interfere. One secondary goal that can often interfere with statement of emotion is *expression of evaluation*. It appears that Joe has the secondary goal of criticizing Minnie for being late. Minnie hears this hidden goal of expressing an evaluation, so she can't hear that Joe is worried. If you embed an evaluation in your statement of emotion, don't expect others to respond the same way they would if you didn't include the evaluation.

In contrast, a secondary goal that supports the statement of emotion is the *gaining of understanding* or, stated another way, *collecting evidence*. When you simply state your emotion, and then listen for the other person's response, you have a chance to learn much about the other person and the situation. If Joe had simply said, "I'm glad you are home, I was worried about you," Minnie might have been able to say (and mean it), "Thanks honey, I'm glad to be home too. I ran into that evil Nate that you don't like; he said he was going to come over for a visit. I had to b.s. him for a while so he wouldn't come over. By the time I was done, the traffic got bad so I was late. How about if I give you one of those special kisses you like?"

Gaining understanding and expression of evaluation are related, but mutually exclusive, activities. You can't do them both at the same time. One way to understand this idea is to be aware that whatever activity we are engaged in, at some level we are always judges. Even when Joe is just telling Minnie he is worried, he is still, at some level, acting like a judge, collecting evidence. When Joe was telling Minnie she was an hour late, he was also acting like a judge — he was evaluating her, declaring her guilty. He acted like he had all the evidence he needed. Judges can't collect evidence and pass a verdict at the same time. So, accept yourself as a judge, judging all that occurs around you, and know there is a time to hear evidence (gain understanding) and a time to state a verdict and sentence.

There is a relationship between combat and the balancing of the two goals — gaining understanding and expression of evaluation — that can cause problems in using FIBRe. In combat, snap decisions, life and death decisions, are made on the basis of something that, in civilian life, is quite superficial, such as clothing. The habit of making quick evaluations was formed under life and death conditions, so it has a tendency to last. That is why it is especially important to get as much practice as possible developing new habits in this area. Combat experiences also may interfere with balanced judgment in another way. Combat experiences lead people to rely on the emotion of anger to avoid the pain of fear and sadness. Angry judges tend to spend too much time finding people guilty (including themselves) and giving out sentences, and not enough time gathering evidence.

It should be mentioned that sometimes people object to the notion that they are judges. Many times these objections come from people who claim to have "low self-esteem," who say they think they are stupid and shouldn't judge (gather evidence and make decisions about) anything. The odd thing is that, even when someone they think is smart comes along and tells them they are smart enough to judge, they *judge* the smart person as wrong and hold to their previous convictions.

Another hidden goal that may get in the way is dominance. Interactions between people can often be rated on the dimension of *affiliation* versus *dominance*. Another way to express this is to say that a communication may have a secondary goal of showing that you are top dog, or it may have the secondary goal of showing that you are partners, working together. If the goal of domination becomes prominent, then it will be more difficult for the other party to hear your primary communication. When Joe pointed at his watch and told Minnie "...look here, it's 11, and you're just now walking in the door," he was giving her the message that he was dominant, that he was in charge of who got home when, and even who looked where (at the watch) when. A communication of dominance in this situation will usually lead a person like Minnie to get angry and not want to be friendly or cooperative, or to not come home at all. You may recognize this dominating type of communication as something you have done unintentionally, by habit, or perhaps you recognize it as something you have done to get people to leave you alone. Practicing FIBRe may help you so you don't use dominating conversation unintentionally, and thus develop better relationships.

Finally, Joe and Minnie might practice FIBRe until they are good enough at it to be more direct with Nate so they don't have to, or want to, b.s. him.

Appendix 2

Substance Abuse

In my experience with clients in my office, usually, when clients are asked to focus on an emergent urge to use an abused substance, and then do EM, the urge simply ends. However, sometimes during the EM, a client may, in imagination, feel he has partaken of the substance, feel the euphoria, move through withdrawal effects, and end with no urge to use. Client reports, as well as therapist observation, of physical movements and expressions consistent with the actual event are similar to what is seen in clients working through trauma experiences. Also supporting the notion that the various aspects of the substance use experience are held in memory networks are substance abusers' reports[1] that they sometimes have dreams that include the "high."

These phenomena, as well as the general clinical experience of myself and others (see discussion below on treatment) support the hypothesis that addictive behavior in its various aspects is held in associative networks and can be processed in the same way as trauma. Just as many reminders of a trauma experience may include partial active repetition of trauma behavior, either in reliving or symbolic repetition (for example, an angry outburst appropriate to the trauma situation, but out of proportion to the current transgression), a number of stimuli may trigger the addictive associative network and lead to addictive behavior. It is hypothesized that processing allows the automatic connection between substance associated stimuli and expectation of substance to be broken. If substance abuse can be conceptualized as partially determined by events triggering the substance use associative network, then treatment may be conceptualized in the four-activity model.

To further relate this substance abuse discussion to earlier discussions, we may note that declarative and nondeclarative memory distinction is relevant to addiction related stimuli and responses. Substance abuse responses may be seen, at least partly, as behavior patterns held in nondeclarative systems, activated by various internal and external cues. (After all, if it were purely a rational–conscious–declarative–information–processing–system decision, no one would use addictive substances to the point of "uncontrollable" self-destructive addiction.) EMDR work with substance abuse associative

---

1. Twelve out of twelve in a recent informal survey of group members in a substance abuse treatment program I conducted.

networks might be conceptualized as integrating the declarative intention that the substance is not to be forthcoming. The conditioned expectation of substance in the accessed situation is then eliminated, just as conditioned fear is eliminated to accessed triggers when a traumatic incident is processed.

When thinking about clients with a primary problem of either trauma reaction or substance abuse, it is helpful to know that a number of research studies show that the relationship between prior trauma and acquiring a substance dependency is strong (Cohen and Densen-Gerber 1982; Grice et al. 1995; Hyer et al. 1991). This suggests that clients whose treatment goals concern PTSD symptoms may have substance abuse issues to be addressed. Of equal importance is the awareness that a client seeking EMDR treatment for substance abuse may have trauma networks that will be triggered by the processing. Shapiro, Sine-Vogel, and Sine (1994) and Popkey (1995) have discussed comprehensive integrative approaches to the use of EMDR with chemical dependency and addiction problems. Readers are referred to their work for treating clients who are currently addicted or not in stable recovery.

In this context, I will emphasize a few points about treatment of clients with substance abuse problems:

1. It is imperative to inform clients that trauma that focuses on trauma or substance abuse (especially if Category 3 activity is involved) may temporarily increase the urge to use. Otherwise, it is impossible for the client to give informed consent.

2. The stronger the addiction network, the more likely it is the client will need to have well-developed Category 4 inhibition activities; these will help to prevent sobriety networks from being overpowered by networks that contain treatment accessed addictive behavior that cannot be fully processed in one session. In this context, the crisis-oriented part of 12-step program activity can be considered Category 4 activity.

3. Work on substance abuse can be conceptualized like work on trauma or any other experience-based problem. Associative networks, including projections of future situations that may lead to the urge to use, must be thoroughly processed for most complete results. Alternative responses to difficult situations must be developed if substance use leading to abuse is not to be chosen again, in the same way the client chose use before becoming dependent or addicted.

Index

A

Accelerated information processing (AIP),
    see also Information processing
    accessing of networks, 18, 24
    experience-based problems, 16
    Humanistic psychotherapeutic position
        homology, 16
    speed of reprocessing, 16, 18, 32
Addiction, EMDR therapy, 137–138
ADHD, *see* Attention deficit hyperactivity
    disorder
AIP, *see* Accelerated information processing
Alpha/theta neurofeedback, PTSD treatment
    efficacy compared with EMDR, 6
Anger management, PTSD treatment efficacy
    compared with EMDR, 7
Antidepressants, use with EMDR, 55–56
Assessment, EMDR
    accessing associative networks, 67–68
    developing solutions, 89–98
    dysfunctional network accessing, 68–69
    negative cognition establishment, 69–73
    overview, 22, 24, 45–46
    personal construct theory, 71–72
    positive cognition introduction, 67–68,
        73–79
    positive schema, *see* Positive schema
    positive vs. preferred cognition, 75–79
    problem and solution
        conceptualization, 74
    processing interference by positive
        cognitions, 77–78
    standard positive cognitions, 77, 89
Attention deficit hyperactivity disorder
    (ADHD), biological component,
    54–55, 56

B

Biofeedback, PTSD treatment efficacy
    compared with EMDR, 3, 4–5

Bipolar affective disorder, biological
    component, 54, 56

C

CBT, *see* Cognitive behavioral therapy
Channel factors, behavioral change, 109
Client education
    goals of therapy, 62
    handout for EMDR, 58–61
    origins of thoughts, feelings, and
        behaviors, 58–60
    psychotherapy overview, 60–61
    rationale, 57
Cognitive behavioral therapy (CBT)
    assessment phase, 46
    negative cognition establishment, 70
Cognitive interweave, EMDR, 73, 80–81
Cognitive processing therapy (CPT), PTSD
    treatment efficacy compared with
    EMDR, 8
Combat veteran, *see* Post-traumatic stress
    disorder
Competence, therapists in EMDR evaluation, 6
Counter-transference, concerns in EMDR
    termination, 124–126
Counting method, facilitating information
    processing, 29
CPT, *see* Cognitive processing therapy

D

Desensitization, EMDR
    aids for eye tracking, 104–105
    distractions, handling, 102, 104
    eye movement mechanics, 101–105
    instructions to patient, 101, 103, 104
    overview, 22, 24, 45, 101
    patient talking effects during
        processing, 103–104
    stopped movement, handling, 105–118

verbal encouragement of patients,
102–103
Desensitization therapy, facilitating
information processing, 30
Dis-identification, positive schema
introduction, 94–95

E

Education, *see* Client education
EMDR, *see* Eye movement desensitization
and reprocessing
Exposure, PTSD treatment efficacy compared
with EMDR, 7–8
Eye movement
activity during arithmetic, 17
aids for eye tracking in EMDR, 104–105
cognitive change reflection, 17
effects as Category 3 activity
heart rate measurements, 37
pain tolerance, 35–36
panic attack, 36
phobias, 36–37, 39
placebo effects, 40, 41
PTSD, 37–38, 39, 40–41
public speaking fear, 38–39
test anxiety, 36
unsupportive studies, 38–41, 43–44
facilitating information processing,
27–28, 29–30, 35–38
mechanics in EMDR, 101–105
sleep and brain functions, 18, 61
suppressive aspects, 17–18, 35
Eye movement desensitization and
reprocessing (EMDR)
attitudes of professionals, 1
controlled studies, 2–6
duration of therapy, 11, 32, 33
outcome, 126
overview, 1
phases, *see* Phases, EMDR
post-traumatic stress disorder,
treatment outcomes compared
with other therapies
combat-related PTSD, 3, 6–7
noncombat-related PTSD, 4, 7–11
surveys of patients and therapists,
5–6, 33
stopped processing, *see* Stopped
movement
substance abuse, 137–138
termination session, 119–121
therapy, 121–125
counter-transference concerns,
124–126

theory, *see* Accelerated information
processing; Four-activity
model

F

FAM, *see* Four-Activity Model
Feelings identification and behavioral
rehearsal group (FIBRe)
applications, 127
comparison to other assertiveness
training, 129–130
focus, 131
forms of behavior, 128
honestly speaking emotions and
thoughts, 131
identification of emotions, 128–129
politely asking for listener attention,
130–131
practical application, 130
practice functions, 130
rationale, 128
request behavior change, 131–132
response, listening, 132
secondary goals and motives, 133–135
troubleshooting, 132–133
vulnerability, 132
FIBRe, *see* Feelings identification and
behavioral rehearsal group
Finger tapping, facilitating information
processing, 41, 42, 43
Flooding
comparison to EMDR, 5–6, 7
facilitating information processing, 30
Forgiveness, role in positive schema
formation, 84, 85, 86
Four-activity model (FAM)
accessing existing information, 25–26
clinical application with EMDR, 51–52
facilitating information processing
abstract activities, 29, 34
auditory stimulation, 30, 43
averse stimuli, 30–31
blinking lights, 42
counting method, 29
definition of activities, 34–35
degrees of processing, 28–29
duration of eye movement, 30
empirical justification in EMDR,
32–35
eye movement, 27–28, 29–30, 35–38
finger tapping, 41, 42, 43
orienting response in mechanism,
31, 44
rapidity of EMDR results, 33–34, 38

For Product Safety Concerns and Information please contact our EU
representative GPSR@taylorandfrancis.com Taylor & Francis Verlag GmbH,
Kaufingerstraße 24, 80331 München, Germany

Printed and bound by CPI Group (UK) Ltd, Croydon, CR0 4YY
08/06/2025
01896998-0017